618.92 G

001949

This book is to be returned on or before the last date stamped below.

A Practical Approach To Clinical Paediatrics

editors

JM Gupta

MBBS (Malaya), MD (Singapore), FRCPE, FRACP, DCH
Visiting Professor of Paediatrics
    University of New South Wales, Sydney, Australia.
Formerly Director Intensive Care Unit
    Prince of Wales Children's Hospital, Sydney, Australia

DW O'Gorman-Hughes

MBBS (Sydney), MD (UNSW), FRACP
Associate Professor of Paediatrics
    University of New South Wales, Sydney, Australia.
Medical Director Children's Leukaemia Cancer Research Centre
    Prince of Wales Children's Hospital, Sydney, Australia

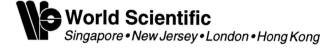
World Scientific
Singapore • New Jersey • London • Hong Kong

Published by

World Scientific Publishing Co. Pte. Ltd.

P O Box 128, Farrer Road, Singapore 912805

USA office: Suite 1B, 1060 Main Street, River Edge, NJ 07661

UK office: 57 Shelton Street, Covent Garden, London WC2H 9HE

Library of Congress Cataloging-in-Publication Data
Gupta, J. M. (Jagdish M.)
    A practical approach to clinical paediatrics / J.M. Gupta, D. W. O'Gorman Hughes.
      p.   cm.
    Includes bibliographical references and index.
    ISBN 9810218494
    1. Paediatrics.   I. Hughes, D. W. O'Gorman.   II. Title.
    [DNLM: 1. Paediatrics.   WS 200 G977p 1995]
RJ45.G95   1995
618.92--dc20
DNLM/DLC
for Library of Congress   95-2640
                                                CIP

British Library Cataloguing-in-Publication Data
A catalogue record for this book is available from the British Library.

For photocopying of material in this volume, please pay a copying fee through the Copyright Clearance Center, Inc., 222 Rosewood Drive, Danvers, MA 01923, USA.

Printed in Singapore.

List of Contributors

EH BATES MSSD (Syd.), FRCS, FRACS, Associate Professor of Paediatrics, University of New South Wales; Paediatric Orthopaedic Surgeon, Prince of Wales Children's Hospital.

HH BODE MD (Saarland), FRACP, DABP, DABPE, Professor of Paediatrics and Head of School University of New South Wales; Director, Prince of Wales Children's Hospital.

TD BOHANE MBBS (Syd.), FRACP, Paediatric Gastroenterologist, Prince of Wales Children's Hospital.

CA CUNNINGHAM OAM, MBBS (Syd.), MRCP (UK), DCH, Developmental Paediatrician; Director, Tumbatin Clinic, Prince of Wales Children's Hospital; Lecturer, University of New South Wales.

BG CURRIE MBBS (Hons) UNSW, FRACS, Paediatric Surgeon, Prince of Wales Children's Hospital; Lecturer, University of New South Wales.

M DUDLEY MBBS (Syd.), BS (Melb.), FRANZCP, Adolescent Psychiatrist, Prince of Wales Children's Hospital.

MA GIBBESON MBBS (UNSW), FRACP, Director, Causalty Services, Prince of Wales Children's Hospital.

T GRATTAN-SMITH MBBS (UNSW), FRACP, Director, Trauma, Prince of Wales Children's Hospital.

JM GUPTA MBBS (Malaya), MD (Singapore), FRCP, FRACP, DCH, Visiting Professor of Paediatrics, University of New South Wales.

J HEADS RNCM Dip Appl Sc (NSG), Dip Teach (NSG), Grad Cert Bio Ethics (IBCLC), MCN (NSW), Clinical Nurse Lactation, Consultant Royal Hospital for Women.

ODH JONES BA (Cant.), MBB (Chir.), MRCP (UK), Senior Lecturer in Paediatrics University of New South Wales, Paediatric Cardiologist, Prince of Wales Children's Hospital.

GM KAINER MBBS (Hons) UNSW, FRACP, Paediatric Nephrologist, Prince of Wales Children's Hospital.

KT MORAN MBBCh (Dublin), BAO, DCH, Dip OBs, FRACP. Medical Director, Child Protection Team, Prince of Wales Children's Hospital.

J MORTON MBBS (Adelaide), FRACGP, FRACP, Head, Respiratory Medicine, Prince of Wales Children's Hospital.

DW O'GORMAN HUGHES MBBS Syd., MD UNSW, FRACP, Associate Professor of Paediatrics, University of New South Wales, Medical Director Children's Leukaemia Cancer Research Centre and Paediatric Haematologist/Oncologist Prince of Wales Children's Hospital.

G TURNER MBBS (St. And.), DSC (UNSW), FRCP, DCH, Associate Professor of Paediatrics, University of New South Wales; Paediatric Geneticist, Prince of Wales Children's Hospital.

JL WALKER MBBS (Syd.), FRACP, Lecturer in Paediatrics, University of New South Wales; Paediatric Endocrinologist, Prince of Wales Children's Hospital.

JB ZIEGLER MBBS (Syd.), FRACP, Associate Professor of Paediatrics, University of New South Wales; Paediatric Immunologist, Prince of Wales Children's Hospital.

Preface

Standard textbooks of Paediatrics describe in detail, normal growth and development, nutrition and nutritional disturbances, infectious diseases and their prevention and diseases affecting various organ systems. Problems in the newborn and inborn errors of metabolism are dealt with separately. While these textbooks meet the needs of the specialist paediatrician and those who need more information on a disease process, they are of limited use to the busy general practitioner. Moreover, children in general practice present to their doctor with symptoms rather than "diseases". This book has been designed to meet the needs of this group of practitioners.

This book is unique in that it deals with problems (symptoms) as they present to the doctor. The problems are approached in a manner that is common practice in clinical paediatrics, namely, obtaining a history followed by physical examination and planning investigations in order to elucidate the diagnosis. General principles of management are discussed but detailed description of diseases and their management is avoided. It is expected that the reader will refer to other textbooks after initial diagnosis.

It is likely that we have inadvertently left out important subjects in the first edition of this book. We will be grateful if readers will indicate to us such omissions so that such subjects may be included in future editions of the book.

November 1995
JM Gupta
DW O'Gorman Hughes

Acknowledgments

We thank Emeritus Professor J Beveridge, Drs H Chilton, M Ferson, H Johnston, I Kennedy, IB Kern, J Mitchell, and B Walder for their helpful suggestions and criticism of this manuscript. Ms M Hope offered valuable suggestions for the chapter on Crying Babies.

This manuscript could not have completed without the valuable help and dedication of Mrs Gail Turner.

Contents

1 Acute Abdominal Pain

Acute abdominal pain in childhood may range from a minor self limiting non-specific illness to a life threatening surgical emergency. It may be the first attack or it may occur in a child who gives a history of recurrent abdominal pain. Age is important when treating childhood abdominal pain because the type of illness, presentation, and pathological conditions differ at various ages. It is also necessary to differentiate conditions that require an operation from those that can be managed medically.

HISTORY

The presenting symptoms in *infants* are irritability and crying which may progress to lethargy and even coma as the illness progresses. Other symptoms which may be present include severe episodic screaming attacks with drawing up of legs due to colic or intussusception (Figs. 1.1 and 1.2), vomiting, diarrhoea, blood and mucus in stools, abdominal distension and features of systemic disease such as fever and rashes.

Toddlers (besides presenting with any of the above symptoms) can indicate that they have abdominal pain. However, they are unable to localise the site of the pain partly due to their inability to communicate and partly due to the nature of the pathological processes in this age group which do not localise the disease process.

In older children, it is possible to determine the location of the pain, its nature, its relation to feeding, its severity and radiation, time and frequency of occurrence and duration; the presence or absence of associated symptoms such as weight loss, fever, vomiting, bloating, diarrhoea, or urinary symptoms; and whether any intermittent illness

1

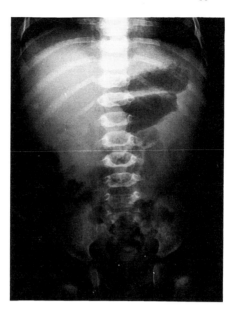

Fig. 1.1 *Intussusception.* Plain X-ray of abdomen shows dilated transverse colon with a rounded filling defect.

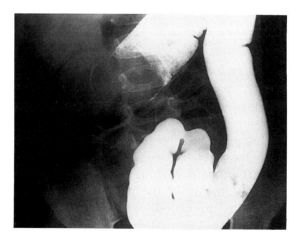

Fig. 1.2 Barium enema shows cup-shaped filling defect from the head of *intussusceptum.*

(past abdominal operations, cystic fibrosis, haemolytic anaemias) or recent trauma has occurred.

In *adolescent girls* a menstrual history should be obtained in order to diagnose conditions such as ectopic pregnancy and dysmenorrhoea. In all cases, information about bowel habit should be obtained.

EXAMINATION

A general physical examination including pulse, respiratory rate, blood pressure, temperature and hydration will be helpful in identifying the ill child and recognising the many systemic conditions which present with acute abdominal pain. Examination of the chest should be carried out carefully, as pneumonia and asthma may occasionally present as abdominal pain. Examination of the scrotum for strangulated hernias and torsion of the testis is mandatory.

In all cases, a careful abdominal examination is necessary. Old operation scars should be noted. Particular attention should be paid to the recognition of the presence of lumps, e.g. sausage shaped lumps in intussusception, "renal lumps" in kidney disease. A loaded colon is often found in patients with constipation. Areas of tenderness should be clearly identified, e.g. tenderness may be localised to the right iliac fossa (in children above the age of 8 years) in appendicitis, salpingitis and mesenteric lymphadenitis; tenderness in the flank and suprapubic region in renal disease; and tenderness in the right hypochondrium in acute cholecystitis.

DIAGNOSIS

There are a number of traps in the diagnosis of acute abdominal pain. Patients with chest infections and asthma with or without respiratory symptoms can present with acute abdominal pain. Children with torsion of the testis may present with acute pain in the right iliac fossa besides the testicular swelling (which the patient may forget to mention). Pain may be the presenting symptom of constipation, worms, diabetic ketoacidosis, lead poisoning (Fig. 1.3), malignant disease, sickle cell

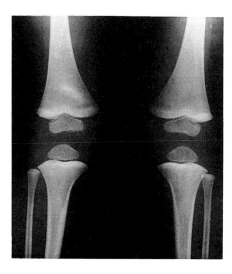

Fig. 1.3 Dense metaphyseal bands seen in *lead poisoning.*

anaemia, porphyria and migraine. Unless a careful history and examination are carried out, the diagnosis may be missed.

Infants suspected of having intussusception will require a barium or air enema which will confirm the diagnosis and may reduce the intussusception.

Acute abdominal pain due to appendicitis may be difficult to distinguish from mesenteric adenitis, as in both conditions the pain may be generalised or localised to the right iliac fossa. History of an acute viral illness with generalised lymphadenitis may help in the diagnosis. Yersinia and campylobacter infection may be confused with regional ileitis; however, a history of weight loss will support the latter diagnosis.

Pain due to renal disease (acute pyelonephritis, pelvi-ureteric junction obstruction) usually starts in the flank before it becomes generalised and may be intermittently colicky. In older girls, the differential diagnosis also includes ectopic pregnancy and salpingitis which can occur without sexual contact and can be confused with appendicitis, ovarian cysts and dysmenorrhoea.

Acute cholecystitis, although uncommon, occurs in children with a history of cystic fibrosis and haemolytic disorders. The pain is usually localised to the right upper quadrant. The pain in acute pancreatitis is severe, central or epigastric and radiates to the back. In these patients, vomiting is a prominent symptom and the patient is often very sick.

MANAGEMENT

The management of infants with acute abdominal pain is complex and requires expert paediatric care. The causes are many and the presentation confusing. They often require urgent resuscitation. Expert advice should be sought early (including by phone) and intravenous fluids should be commenced.

In older children, the diagnosis may be obvious from the history and physical examination but often it is obscure and early involvement of a paediatric specialist is helpful in directing tests and management. Often the only decision that needs to be made is whether the child needs to have an operation or not, with the exact diagnosis unclear until laparotomy or further tests are performed. It is more important to recognise and resuscitate the child and to obtain expert advice early than it is to pursue an exact diagnosis with multiple investigations.

2 Recurrent Abdominal Pain

Recurrent abdominal pain is one of the commonest conditions seen in general practice. However, a child with recurrent abdominal pain may have an acute presentation and an acute presentation may be the first episode of recurrent abdominal pain.

HISTORY

The physician should inquire about the timing, quality, location, radiation, severity and cause of the pain episodes. Information about events surrounding the initial attack and those associated with subsequent attacks should be explored. It should also be determined to what extent pain disrupts normal activity (school, play, sleep) and the measures that relieve or exacerbate it (position, food, medications, rest). It is also important to determine whether the episodes occur irregularly, in clusters and at particular times of the day. It is preferable to obtain this information from the child and the parents separately.

Besides obtaining information about the pain, questions should be asked to determine whether there is any particular cause for concern, e.g. there may be a fear of a specific disease process such as cancer or some other disease a friend or relative may be suffering from.

Most children with recurrent abdominal pain do not have an organic cause. Therefore a history directed towards development, environmental relationships and family dynamics is important. Chronic constipation due to stool retention as a result of emotional problems is one of the commonest causes of recurrent abdominal pain — hence a history of bowel habit is very important.

Information should also be obtained for other gastrointestinal symptoms such as nausea, anorexia, diarrhoea (with or without blood). Patients with recurrent abdominal pain due to inflammatory bowel disease will have a history of weight loss, poor growth, delay in onset of puberty and may have joint, skin or eye symptoms as a result of the complications of the disease. Children with malignant disease appear unwell, have lost weight, and may have intermittent fever and abdominal masses.

Family history is very important, not only in terms of various diseases such as peptic ulcer disease, inflammatory bowel disease, coeliac disease, gastro-oesophageal reflux, but also whether there is a family history of recurrent abdominal pain in childhood. The other known organic diseases that often run in families are migraine, irritable bowel and diverticular disease.

EXAMINATION

Usually there is no abnormality on examination in these children although at times there may be evidence of faecal retention. The physician should focus on the child as to whether he or she is anxious, depressed, or over playing the symptoms or the signs, and whether there is abdominal tenderness which is focal or generalised. The child should be asked to pinpoint the site of the pain — if it is vague or localised to the umbilicus, it is almost certainly non-organic. The physician should palpate for masses in the abdomen and look for evidence of constipation. There may be evidence of inflammatory bowel disease (sinuses and fissures in the perineum). A general physical examination should include measurement of blood pressure, examination of fundi and evidence of lead poisoning (anaemia, blue line on the gums). A rectal examination is important to ensure there is no significant stool retention.

MANAGEMENT

The age of the patient must be taken into account when making an aetiological diagnosis of recurrent abdominal pain. Infants and toddlers are likely to have organic causes until proven otherwise, whereas school-age children are more likely to have non-organic causes. The diagnosis of non-organic recurrent abdominal pain (dysfunctional pain or psychogenic pain) must be made on the history and physical examination and not on the basis of absence of organic disease.

In the absence of clues to a diagnosis, analysis of urine (sugar, protein, microscopic examination and culture) and stool (occult blood, ova, cysts and parasites and culture for yersinia), full blood count (including peripheral smear and reticulocyte count) and ESR should be undertaken. In most cases, further investigations are rarely necessary if recurrent abdominal pain is the only symptom.

The most important aspect of management is to assure the family that the child does not have any serious disease. If there is evidence of stool retention, this should be treated. It is important not to request "one more test" to ensure that the child does not have a disease process, as it will only reinforce the parent's belief that the child has some organic disease. Sometimes a plain abdominal film may be helpful in the diagnosis when chronic faecal retention is suspected.

3 Child Physical Abuse (Non-Accidental Injury in Infants and Young Children)

There are some inflicted injuries where there is no doubt about the diagnosis, e.g. stab wounds. This discussion concerns injuries where the diagnosis may not be apparent initially.

HISTORY

In inflicted injury, the history given is rarely an accurate one. The doctor is alerted to this fact later by one of the following circumstances:

1. The injuries are clearly incompatible with the history.
2. There is confusion about the manner of injury which may be cleared up when the history is reviewed with the caretaker.
3. The history changes as the caretaker adapts it to conform with information learned from the doctors.
4. Children who present unconscious or in severe shock may have been abused. The child may have a severe head injury and/or severe abdominal trauma. The history given will rarely account for the serious nature of the injuries or there may be no eyewitness account.
5. Certain injuries diagnosed by special studies are virtually diagnostic of child abuse, regardless of the history.

EXAMINATION

Major Head Injury

Important parts of the examination are documentation of:

(i) external trauma to the head, abdomen, limbs and trunk including bruises or burns.
(ii) examination of the retina for haemorrhages. The presence of retinal haemorrhages may be good evidence of a shake impact injury.

   The literature supports the view that falls from a short distance do not cause major injuries. The forces needed to cause such injuries arise from long falls or from motor vehicle accidents.

Abdominal Injuries

There may be no external evidence of injury to the abdomen despite severe damage to internal organs. The child may present acutely (in shock) or subacutely (over a period of days). The trauma is usually inflicted by a blow to the abdomen and is similar to that seen in children who are run over by motor vehicles. The most frequently injured organs are the liver, the spleen, the duodenum, the proximal jejunum, the distal ileum, the pancreas and the mesentery. Obviously, other organs may be injured.

Skin Injury

Bruising over bony prominences is usually accidental, e.g. tibiae, forearms, forehead, maxilla or mandible. Bruising over the cheek, the buttocks, the genital or perianal area is suspicious of inflicted injury. Handmarks or patterned bruising in the form of an object need no further elucidation. Bruising on very young infants always arouses suspicion whereas single bruises on infants just walking are common. Multiple bruises, particularly of varying ages, are suspicious of inflicted injury.

Burns

Cigarette burns may be recognised by their circular shape and size (but should not be confused with bullous impetigo lesions) (Fig. 3.1). Occasionally, they may be accidental, but in this case they are not deep, and are usually single and not circular.

Pattern burns are produced by specific hot objects being brought in contact with the skin. Usually if children have brushed against these unintentionally they are likely to be 1st or 2nd degree burns and are usually deeper and of more severe degree on one edge of the burn. Caretakers ought to be able to give a reasonable reconstruction in these cases. The location of the burn, the pattern and the age of the child should help differentiate inflicted from accidental injury. It may be necessary to visit the house to verify the events.

Immersion burns are often severe and assessment should include information about water temperature, placement of taps, depth of water and the position of the child in the water. The presence of splash marks (more likely in accidental burns) vs. glove or stocking distribution is helpful in determining whether a body part was forcefully immersed. Second or third degree burns are likely to have been inflicted, whereas first degree burns may occur if a child accidentally immerses a hand or foot in hot water.

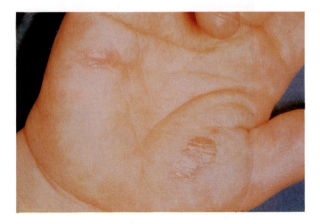

Fig. 3.1 *Child Physical Abuse.* Cigarette burns.

Tap water scalds which are deliberate are like accidental spills but they involve the buttocks, legs and perineum more frequently.

Children who pull containers of hot liquid from tables or stoves have a characteristic pattern of burns which is quite different from that seen in immersion burns.

Abrasions and Lacerations

Inflicted injuries must be differentiated from the small abrasions that young babies can inflict on themselves from their nails before the age of 3 months. Commonly, inflicted injuries are caused by buckles or other objects and may have a characteristic shape (Fig. 3.2). Strap marks, loop marks or circumferential marks from tying may be seen. A hairbrush may leave punctate bruises.

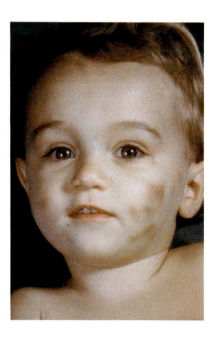

Fig. 3.2 *Child Physical Abuse.* Finger pressure marks on cheeks.

Mouth Lesions

In infants a tear in the frenulum of the lip is caused usually by ramming a bottle into the baby's mouth. In toddlers who run with a bottle in the mouth, this injury may occur accidentally. Bruising of the palate may occur in the same way. Burns of the palate may occur with bottles heated in a microwave and may indicate neglect or abuse. Injuries to the teeth may occur accidentally or as a result of blows to the mouth. Toddlers more commonly sustain these injuries in falls.

Fractures

A fracture may present acutely or an old fracture may be discovered as part of an assessment for another reason, e.g. rib fractures on chest X-ray (Fig. 3.3) or multiple fractures on skeletal survey (Fig. 3.4).

A knowledge of how different fractures commonly occur, the child's age and developmental stage and a good history of the incident help in making an assessment. It may be necessary to undertake a bone scan to look for injuries which are difficult to detect on conventional X-rays.

Fractures of the clavicle may be due to birth trauma in the newborn. Otherwise all fractures in children who are not yet walking, who are not affected by bone disease, and who have not been involved in a documented motor vehicle accident, should be considered non-accidental. A fall from 1 metre onto a hard surface can result in a linear parietal skull fracture with no intracranial pathology and no retinal haemorrhage. Fractures of the metaphysis, the so-called "bucket-handle" or "corner" fractures are almost diagnostic of abuse because of the mechanism of injury, as are rib fractures in infancy.

Fractures of the midshaft of the femur are almost always inflicted in non-ambulant infants. It can be more difficult to make an assessment after this age and an isolated femoral fracture cannot confirm a diagnosis of child abuse.

Fractures of the distal radius and ulna result from falls on the outstretched hand.

Multiple fractures of different ages are either due to abuse or bone disease such as osteogenesis imperfecta, scurvy, osteoporosis, malignant disease, copper deficiency due to malabsorption in low birth weight infants, diet or excess loss as in dialysis.

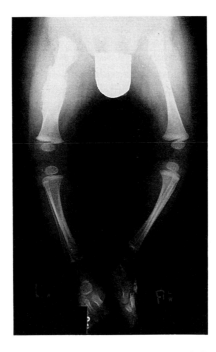

Fig. 3.3 Healing mid-shaft spiral fracture of femur and "bucket handle" fracture of lower left tibia in a 6-month-old infant with *child physical abuse.*

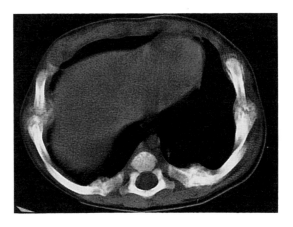

Fig. 3.4 CT scan shows multiple rib fractures at different stages of healing consistent with *child physical abuse.*

Suffocation

It may be impossible to distinguish suffocation at autopsy from asphyxia due to some natural cause such as sudden infant death syndrome. Repetitive suffocation may be recognised before severe damage occurs.

Munchausen Syndrome by Proxy

This refers to children whose mothers invent stories of illness in the child and who may substantiate the stories by fabricating false signs.

There is a spectrum of parents ranging from those with needless anxiety about trivial illnesses to those who fabricate physical signs.

Warning signs are unexplained, prolonged, rare illnesses; symptoms and signs present only in association with mother's presence; frequent treatment failures; and the presence of similar symptoms in other members of the family.

There is no definite psychiatric diagnosis for these parents but there is frequently significant psychological morbidity for the child. Children may be subjected to invasive investigations and harmful treatment. Accidental deaths have been reported.

MANAGEMENT

In many Australian states it is the law that suspected child abuse and neglect be reported to a statutory authority which has responsibility for the protection of the child. Criminal proceedings may ensue against the responsible adult through police action. Doctors should make sure that their documentation of injuries is clear and explains the nature, mechanism and timing of the injury as well as the consequences for the child.

The most important part of treatment is to stop the abuse, and to prevent serious injuries to the child. Initially this can be done by admitting the child to hospital for "investigations". Further action such as fostering or permanent removal of the child from the home will depend on family relationships (isolation, lack of support, violence towards the mother, and drug and alcohol abuse by parents).

In many cases, a skeletal survey may be necessary to establish a diagnosis. Haematological studies may be necessary to exclude a bleeding disorder. Patients in coma or shock may have head or abdominal injuries and will require further investigations (ultrasound, CT scan) to diagnose internal injuries requiring specific treatment.

Long term management requires the intervention of social workers and mental health professionals. The abuse must be acknowledged and the aim is to make parents more emotionally responsive to their children's needs so that the family has a more adaptive method of functioning. Some families are untreatable and in such cases, fostering and sometimes permanent removal of the child is necessary.

4 Child Sexual Abuse

Doctors find making a diagnosis of sexual abuse difficult for several reasons: the mode of presentation may be unfamiliar to them, there is often inadequate training in examining normal female children's genitalia, or they are reluctant to countenance such an impalatable possibility.

If they consider the diagnosis then they face further hurdles in obtaining the history in an accurate and unbiased way, performing a competent examination and understanding the complexity of laboratory evidence which may assist in making the diagnosis. Add to this, the social and legal ramifications of the diagnosis and it is not surprising that most thoughtful professionals become anxious when faced with the possibility of child sexual abuse.

HISTORY

These children present in a variety of ways depending on the relationship to the person perpetrating the abuse.

Child abuse by strangers is relatively uncommon. In such cases the children usually tell their parents who in turn may seek help. Those abused in institutions (day care, school), are usually under considerable pressure not to communicate with their parents. In such cases, many children are involved and the situation comes to light after one or two of the children tell their parents. The majority of sexual abuse (30–50%) is perpetrated by family members (17% by step-fathers) — these children present with psychosomatic complaints, inappropriate sexual behaviour for age, non-specific genital symptoms, sexually transmitted diseases and pregnancy. Finally, sexual abuse may present with a history of sexual assault.

The history should be taken by experienced personnel who should be able to establish a rapport with the child. A supportive parent can be helpful to a young child during the interview but non-supportive parents and possible perpetrators should never be present at initial interviews. Most children above the age of 3 years can recall and tell about sexual abuse and are no more likely than adults to distort, fantasise or otherwise incorrectly report past events. The use of anatomically correct dolls sometimes allows children to express past events that they would otherwise have difficulty in telling. Drawings by the child serve a similar function. False statements from young children in their interviews about sexual abuse are relatively rare. It is more likely that children may not describe abuse when it is present.

Besides obtaining the details about the abuse, the interviewer should ask questions about pain or bleeding, urinary frequency, desire to defaecate, taste (if appropriate) and about how the child felt during the abuse.

PHYSICAL EXAMINATION

It is important that the child should be given an explanation about the physical examination and if possible, the child should choose the gender of the examining physician as many female victims have a generalised fear of men. The physician should have special training (know normal female anatomy, techniques for exposing the hymen) and experience in examining children for sexual abuse. Many centres have a protocol for these examinations and if so, then it should be followed.

Before undertaking examination of the vulva and anal area, the physician should carry out a general physical examination. The child should be in the supine position normally or in the knee/chest position if confirmation of suspicious hymenal findings make this necessary. Examination of the anus is important to look for evidence of abnormal sphincter tone, discharge, scars or distortion. Vesicles or warts may be found in the perineal and vulval regions.

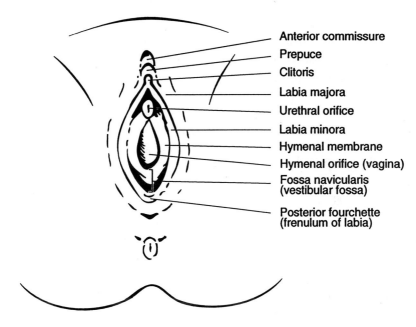

Fig. 4.1 Anatomy of the vulva.

MANAGEMENT

In all cases, cultures should be taken for *N. gonorrhoeae* and *chlamydia*. Serological tests for syphilis may be necessary. In the presence of vesicles, virological confirmation of Herpes simplex is necessary. Virological confirmation of the diagnosis of warts is difficult though a Pap smear may be useful. In cases of suspected rape, additional laboratory tests are needed and specimens from the victim's clothing, hair and body are required. Microscopical examination of vaginal, oral or rectal secretions for sperms is also essential. Post pubertal victims may need pregnancy testing.

Good records are important for medicolegal reasons and findings and conclusions should be described simply.

It is important to talk to parents and adolescents about the examination findings and to emphasise normality and rapidity of healing. A crisis is inevitable in a family in which sexual abuse is suspected. It is important that such a family be assessed quickly by a social worker and/or a mental health professional. In most Australian states it is also a legal requirement that the suspicion should be reported to a statutory authority.

The reason for further evaluation of a child and family is to validate the allegation, undertake a forensic evaluation and to determine the impact of the abuse on the child and family. It may be necessary to assess the degree of future risk to the child. Ongoing treatment involves individual, group and family therapy.

5 Separation Anxiety

Separation anxiety may present clinically at any time from infancy to adolescence, but its significance varies with age. Some degree of separation anxiety is normal later in infancy. Separation anxiety also may be seen in relation to separations in kindergarten and first grade, with distressing events in childhood (hospitalisation), and often around the time of commencement of high school. Separation anxiety is judged to be clinically significant when the child is older, and when symptoms are severe, exceed normal developmental limits, and cause serious distress or impairment, e.g. also affect peer relationships.

HISTORY

The duration and quality of the anxiety in infancy will vary considerably with the security of the attachment between the infant and mother. Securely attached infants are calmed by contact with their mothers when they are separated or otherwise under stress, whereas anxiously attached infants may be ambivalent toward their mothers or avoid them at times of separation. The latter (anxious-ambivalent or anxious-avoidant) groups of infants are unable to use their mothers as a secure base from which to explore, and their mothers often have difficulties in being appropriately responsive to, and may be rejecting of, their infant's care-eliciting.

Children with separation anxiety are afraid of any separation from principal attachment figures and/or familiar surroundings. They may refuse to sleep over with friends, to take school trips or to go on errands, may show distress on separation, and may have nightmares with separation themes. They may have fears of losing their family, or death or other disaster. In a variant of this, the child refuses to attend school and expresses anxiety in association with school attendance. Somatic symptoms (abdominal pain, palpitations, headache) are often prominent and may be the presenting complaints. These symptoms often reach a crescendo after weekends and holidays, or before school, and may disappear when the time for leaving for school has passed.

There may be a family history of separation anxiety and other anxiety or psychiatric disorders (e.g. post-natal depression) and a history of losses or other negative events that may have acted as triggers. A secondary pattern of over-protection may have emerged in family relationships in response to these events.

EXAMINATION

During the examination, the child may be anxious, depressed, or angry and one or both parents may be anxious or depressed. The parent-child interaction may reveal difficulties with separation, e.g. leaving the child in the waiting room, and there may be heightened responsiveness within the family to each other's cues observed within the session.

DIAGNOSIS

If separation anxiety begins shortly after a stressor (e.g. parental separation and divorce, a family move or changing schools) and lasts less than six months, a diagnosis of adjustment disorder with anxious mood may be given. Children and adolescents with severe separation anxiety may also have co-existent panic disorder (characterised by panic attacks similar to those in adults). Children with an overanxious disorder are affected with concerns about competence (e.g. examinations, meeting deadlines), approval (from peers, adults), appropriateness of past behaviour and the future. They may also have physical symptoms such as headaches and abdominal pain with no physical basis. Fears are very common in childhood and when a specific fear is associated with avoidance behaviour and results in functional or social impairment, then the diagnosis of phobia is warranted. Depression should also be considered and frequently co-occurs with separation anxiety and school refusal. Separation anxiety may also present in the context of an overwhelming trauma with post-traumatic symptoms.

MANAGEMENT

With younger children, treatment may be relatively simple. The diagnosis and nature of the disorder are explained to the parents and child, and the potential contagion of anxiety within families. Children need to experience separations in order to discover that their fears of harm coming to themselves or their attachment figures are unfounded. Parents will need to be reassured, and to reassure the child that the child will be all right. Separations are then undertaken at the natural times and the child is given praise and possibly other rewards for doing so.

If school refusal is part of the presenting problem, treatment with younger children will usually involve getting the child back to school as soon as possible. This requires the family, the school and the treatment team to work together to arrive at a united and well planned strategy. An assessment ensures that the child is capable of returning to school (almost always the case), and considers factors within the child and family that are perpetuating the problem, as well as the strengths that can be used to support the child's self-esteem. Any measures that can make the school environment less stressful or can support the child are implemented. The child is informed of the plan, which has a date for the proposed return to school, and "fall-back" positions should be worked out beforehand should the child fail to get out of bed or leave the house. The least desirable alternative will be remaining at or returning home. Firm, calm handling and a united approach is usually effective in acute cases in effecting return to school. Education departments often have home-school liaison officers who assist in this process.

Psychotherapy is the mainstay of the treatment of separation anxiety. It will often have a family focus, but may be augmented by work with the child and/or the parents. Parental over-protective or over-anxious responses will be addressed in family or parental therapy, and further individual treatment for parental psychiatric disorders may be indicated.

Individual therapy for the child directed at the child's anxieties and conflicts (which may be unconscious) may also be useful, especially if the condition is chronic or affects many aspects of the child's life and functioning. As noted, behavioural approaches may be useful in dealing with factors in the environment that may be reinforcing the child's symptoms (e.g. teacher and parent responses). Pharmacotherapy with sedative-hypnotic agents is usually contraindicated with anxiety disorders in childhood, because they are ineffective in addressing the central problems (which are generally environmental and psychological, rather than individual and biological in origin), and pharmacotherapy also often gives the impression that there is a magic "fix". They may be used in the very short term (i.e. days only) for severe anxiety that is related to a situational stress. Antidepressants have been used in children and adolescents with panic attacks.

More refractory cases of separation anxiety may need to be referred to a child psychiatrist. As well as the above measures, hospitalisation and medication may also be necessary and will need to be carefully negotiated with the parents, since the separation may also be a major difficulty for them. Where school refusal is more chronic, the child is usually older, more anxious, depressed and panicky; the parents may also be psychiatrically ill. A period of psychotherapy for the child or parents may be required to facilitate the child's return to school, possibly aided by treatment in a daypatient or inpatient unit. Imipramine has been described as being of potential value in addition to these supportive and behavioural measures, particularly if there are panic attacks; but its efficacy is not proven in clinical trials, and since it may be cardiotoxic and have at times led to sudden death, it should be used with appropriate precautions and warnings.

School refusal in adolescence is often more difficult to treat, and has a poorer prognosis. It is harder to persuade the adolescent to attend and may be an indication of more serious pathology.

6 Breastfeeding Problems

HISTORY

Breastfeeding problems may occur while the mother is still in the maternity hospital or may emerge after she has been discharged home. Common problems are difficulty in attachment, integrity of the nipple or areola and perceived low milk supply. The mother should be asked about her general health (complications of pregnancy, delivery and puerperium), her diet and her ability to rest and sleep. The exact nature of the feeding difficulty has to be determined accurately (e.g. mother feels pain on feeding or the baby refuses to feed and cries when placed on the breast). It is also necessary to determine her attitude towards breastfeeding and the advice she has received from other people in prenatal counselling or advice from relatives and friends. The attitude of the immediate family members such as the husband, mother, mother-in-law will also determine whether breastfeeding is likely to be successful. The baby's urinary output and weight gain will reflect the volume of milk intake. Frequent small loose green stools indicate inadequate milk intake.

PHYSICAL EXAMINATION

Examination involves that of the mother, baby and feeding process. The mother's breasts should be examined for the presence of lumps, tenderness, redness and the nipples and areola for skin integrity (damaged nipples, infection — thrush, dermatitis). Mothers with inflexible nipples may have difficulty with breastfeeding.

Examination of the baby includes assessment of maturity and ensuring that it is able to suck. Babies with respiratory, cardiac and neurological abnormalities may present as feeding difficulties. The only localised structural abnormalities which may interfere with breastfeeding are an abnormal palate (cleft palate, high arched palate) or choanal atresia.

In the evaluation of breastfeeding problems, the baby needs to be watched while feeding. Important observations that need to be made include how the mother holds the baby, the behaviour of baby during feeds, efficiency of let-down reflex which is indicated by change in baby's sucking rhythm from short shallow sucks to a deep rhythmical suck and swallow pattern. Some mothers will have a tingling sensation during the let-down reflex.

MANAGEMENT

General measures include good diet, rest, sleep and encouragement of the mother in her style of mothering in order to build her confidence. Encouraging contact with support groups like the Nursing Mothers Association of Australia, is helpful. Sore nipples have to be treated with appropriate oral analgesics and in extreme cases it may be necessary to express the milk and feed the baby until such time as the nipples are healed. Breast infections will require local moist heat to affected area before feeds, oral analgesics and broad spectrum antibiotics for 10 days. Breast infection is not a contraindication for continuing breastfeeding.

During the feed, the mother should be comfortable, the baby's chest should be next to hers and she should support the weight of the baby in her arm. When the baby's cheek touches the breast, it will elicit the rooting reflex. The nipple, areola and underlying breast tissue are drawn to the baby's mouth. During feeding, the baby's chin should be tucked well into the breast allowing the nose to stay clear in order to prevent obstruction to breathing. The baby's cheeks will be full during sucking (not pinched in) and there should be no loud clicking. Particular attention should be paid to ensure that the mother has an adequate let-down reflex. For the mother, the experience should be pain free. At the completion of the feed, the nipple's shape will be slightly elongated.

Damage to the nipple, indicated by stress lines, blanching or squashing, is due to poor positioning.

There are no fixed rules about the duration and frequency of feeding. However, in order to ensure that there is no damage to the nipples, the baby should be sucking on the areola rather than the nipple. The baby should be allowed to spontaneously terminate sucking (rather than taking it off after a designated period) on the first breast to ensure complete drainage before offering the other breast. This allows the baby to obtain the hind milk (rich in fat) which will help in satiety and nutrition.

Delayed milk let-down can be related to nipple damage, as pain and fear trigger the release of adrenalin and noradrenaline which impede the action of oxytocin. In such cases, adequate analgesia is essential for successful breastfeeding.

Mothers with inflexible nipples may be helped to breastfeed by the use of a silicon nipple shield.

Breast refusal is usually temporary and often is a symptom of some other underlying problem such as an unwell baby or mother. It can also be due to confusion caused to the baby when the cheek away from the breast is touched in an effort to help the mother to put the baby on the breast. The baby turns towards the helper as a result of the rooting reflex.

Adequate milk intake can be best assessed by weighing the baby frequently. In most cases weighing the baby weekly is adequate though in some cases it may be necessary to weigh the baby twice a week. Test weighing is inappropriate and will only result in further maternal anxiety and diminution of milk supply. Weight gain in babies is variable from week to week and though some babies may gain 150–300 grams a week, a gain of 100 grams a week may be adequate in others.

In the rare cases of inadequate milk supply (poor weight gain), increasing the frequency of feeds will help to alleviate the problem as sucking is the best stimulus for milk production. Some mothers can be helped by "supply lines" also referred to as "supplemental nursing system".

7 Does the Child Have Cancer?

The incidence of childhood cancer is about one in 550 under the age of 15 years which implies an annual incidence of about 1 in 8000 children. With an overall cure rate between 60% and 70% in many developed countries, a great deal of energy has been devoted to improving the relief of symptoms and cure rate over the past few years.

HISTORY

The presenting symptoms and signs may be multiple and variable, but taken in context may lead to strong suspicion of an underlying malignancy. Some of these features include a lump, pain, pallor, a limp, abnormal gait or difficulty in walking, headaches and vomiting, fever, fatigue, weight loss and anorexia, bruising, and respiratory difficulty.

1. *A lump or lumps*: These may be detected in the neck, abdomen, limbs or head. Characteristically they are painless and firm. Abdominal masses may cause pain, but if due to malignancy are usually not tender and are firm to hard in texture.
2. *Pain* in malignant disease is especially likely to occur in the abdomen or at a peripheral site such as in bones or joint areas. It is often very intense, may occur suddenly at night and may settle abruptly after analgesics (such as paracetamol) and recur a day or several days later. It is not usually related to activity. The pain in limbs may be due to diffuse marrow infiltration as in leukaemia or disseminated neuroblastoma, or to a more localised bone tumour such as osteogenic or Ewing's sarcoma, or to joint involvement or to nerve root irritation as in spinal or pelvic infiltration.

3. **Pallor** due to anaemia, especially in an unwell child and of recent origin, should arouse strong suspicion of a malignancy such as leukaemia, lymphoma or neuroblastoma infiltrating bone marrow.

4. **Fever.** A documented history of fever exceeding 38.5°C over a period of several weeks is moderately common in cases of leukaemia, lymphoma and Wilms' tumour and may be the dominant feature.

5. **General symptoms** such as *fatigue, weight loss* or *loss of appetite* occur in many diseases but malignancy should be suspected if no other obvious cause (such as infection or malabsorption) can be found.

6. **A limp or abnormal gait** may be due to several causes including injury, infection such as septic arthritis or osteomyelitis, soft tissue inflammatory disease such as synovitis, myositis or rheumatoid arthritis, or from spinal or nerve involvement or compression. Malignant disease causes symptoms by local infiltration causing pain or restricted movement or by nerve compression at a spinal or peripheral level. Examples are bone infiltration (leukaemia, lymphoma, neuroblastoma, bone sarcoma), or soft tissue lesions (soft tissue sarcoma) and tumours impinging on the spinal cord (especially from neuroblastoma, rhabdomyosarcoma, lymphoma, or spinal cord primary tumours). The gait may be atalgic or may be due to neurological deficits. It is important to enquire about motor weakness and disturbances of bowel or bladder function. Constipation or dysuria for example may be due to nerve compression by a paraspinal tumour.

7. **Headaches and vomiting,** especially if occurring in the mornings after awakening are features strongly implicating raised intracranial pressure and may be due to intracranial tumours or neuroleukaemia. Symptoms may appear for a few days then disappear for a while and recur. The child's blood pressure should be measured and the fundi examined for papilloedema.

8. **Respiratory difficulties.** A history of fatigue exertional dyspnoea, noisy breathing ("wheezing" or snoring) and orthopnoea, particularly if occurring in rapid sequence should alert the clinician to the possibility of mediastinal compression due to tumour, which may be caused by lymphoma, leukaemia or teratoma.

9. **Bleeding** may be manifest from mucosal, subcutaneous or cutaneous sites. In malignant disease the most likely cause is thrombocytopenia,

secondary to marrow infiltration but occasionally local gastro-intestinal lesions may produce haematemesis or malaena and renal lesions may cause haematuria.

EXAMINATION

The height, weight and head circumference should be measured and the child assessed for evidence of recent weight loss, pallor, bruising, visible abnormalities of gait and for lumps. In the abdomen, evidence of distension, hepatosplenomegaly or abdominal masses should be sought and if present, it should be determined whether the masses are lateral (as in Wilms' tumour, splenomegaly, hepatoblastoma, neuroblastoma, leukaemia) or central (as in lymphoma, neuroblastoma, rhabdomyo-sarcoma or germ cell tumour). Painless testicular enlargement may be the presenting sign of testicular tumours.

In the thorax, the respiratory rate, evidence of mediastinal or pleural dullness and altered breath sounds should be assessed. In the neck, supraclavicular and cervical lymph nodes may be enlarged. Abnormalities on examination of the head may include cranial nerve palsies, proptosis, lumps on the scalp and papilloedema. Lumps or swellings in the limbs may indicate a site of a primary or secondary tumour.

MANAGEMENT

Rapid and important decisions are required if the child is ill or pale and life threatening problems include acute respiratory obstruction, impending paraplegia, bleeding or severe anaemia. In the vast majority of cases, investigations are required to establish a definitive diagnosis before treatment is commenced.

8 Coma

The unconscious child usually requires urgent admission to hospital, but should be assessed prior to transfer in case emergency treatment is required.

PHYSICAL EXAMINATION

1. Assess level of coma. How rousable is the child?
2. Check adequacy of airways, breathing, circulation (pulse and blood pressure) and state of hydration. Some urgent supportive measures may be required.
3. Check for any diagnostic clinical clues on quick examination such as:

Signs & Symptoms	Likely Cause
Acidotic breathing	Dehydration, gastroenteritis, diabetic ketoacidosis, poisons
Ketones on breath	Diabetes mellitus
Purpuric rash	Meningococcal septicaemia
Rapid weak pulse	Dehydration and poisoning, septic shock
Sweating	Hypoglycaemia

Cyanosis	Airway obstruction, peripheral circulatory failure
Local neurological signs such as hemiparesis; altered reflexes; unequal, dilated or fixed pupils	Intracranial haemorrhage, injury, mass lesions, bacterial meningitis
Fundal haemorrhages or papilloedema	Intracranial bleeding and swelling

4. HISTORY

Features	Possible Cause
Onset — sudden (hours)	Bleeding, injury, hypoglycaemia, meningococcal septicaemia, ingestion of poisons
Onset — slower (day/days)	Diabetic ketoacidosis, bacterial meningitis
Vomiting	Drug or poison ingestion, acute viral infection, meningitis, intracranial mass lesions, diabetic ketoacidosis
Diarrhoea	Poisoning, gastroenteritis
Polyuria, polydipsia	Diabetes mellitus
Oliguria	Renal disease, dehydration
Prolonged fasting or poor intake for 1 or more days	Hypoglycaemia

Previous headaches, irritability or confusion	Bacterial meningitis, encephalitis, hypertensive encephalopathy, intracranial haemorrhage
Previous head injury	Intracranial haemorrhage (extradural, subdural haemorrhages), cerebral oedema
Recent convulsions and abnormal movements	Post ictal coma; think also of hypoglycaemia

MANAGEMENT

In general, as little time as possible should be wasted in sending the child urgently to hospital, accompanied by a doctor whenever possible.

However the following measures are important.

1. Maintain airways and oxygen.
2. If the child is hypovolaemic an intravenous drip should be inserted rapidly.
3. If hypoglycaemia is suspected, collect blood for glucose level and give intravenous dextrose.
4. If meningococcal septicaemia is suspected, give intravenous or intramuscular penicillin (1 million units). If possible collect blood culture first.
5. If fitting occurs, control may be achieved by intravenous diazepam.

9 Congestive Cardiac Failure

HISTORY

Presenting features include feeding difficulties, failure to thrive, rapid weight gain, breathlessness, tachypnoea, tachycardia, generalised sweating especially during feeding and crying, "shock", pale looking unwell child and cyanosis. Oedema is rare in infants though it may occur in older children who may even have generalised anasarca.

PHYSICAL EXAMINATION

In infants, signs include shock-like state — low pulse volume, low blood pressure and pallor, tachypnoea with or without recession, rales and rhonchi, cardiac enlargement, tachycardia, gallop rhythm, enlarged liver. Jugular venous pressure is difficult to assess in infants. Other signs will depend on aetiology, e.g. murmurs in structural heart lesions, raised blood pressure and delayed femoral pulses in coarctation of aorta, and cyanosis in right to left shunts.

INVESTIGATIONS

ECG to evaluate rate, rhythm, axis, cardiac enlargement, ischemia.
Chest X-ray to establish heart size, pulmonary vasculature.
Echocardiogram to outline structural anatomy.
Cardiac catheterisation to establish accurately pressures in cardiac chambers.

DIAGNOSIS

The main causes of heart failure are increased volume or pressure loads and myocardial dysfunction.

Excess volume loads occur due to left to right shunts and valvular incompetence. In the premature infant, patent ductus arteriosus and large ventricular septal defects can cause heart failure but in the full term infant these lesions do not produce heart failure until after 6 weeks of age because it takes a longer time for the pulmonary vascular resistance to fall. However, large left to right shunts (e.g. endocardial cushion defect, arteriovenous fistulas, complex anatomic lesions such as truncus arteriosus and transposition) can present with heart failure in the term infant at any age. Other causes of excessive volume loads are a large infusion of blood or fluid and impaired renal function.

Pressure loads are due to obstructive lesions which include severe aortic stenosis, coarctation of aorta and total anomalous pulmonary venous drainage. In the immediate newborn period, severe pulmonary hypertension causes right sided congestive cardiac failure.

Myocardial causes of heart failure include myocarditis, cardiomyopathy, endocardial fibroelastosis, anomalous left coronary artery. These are rare in neonates who are more likely to have heart failure due to metabolic disturbances such as asphyxia, acidosis and hypoglycaemia. Other causes of myocardial dysfunction include paroxysmal tachycardia, congenital heart block and polycythaemia.

MANAGEMENT

Structural abnormalities require surgical correction other than patent ductus arteriosus in the newborn (especially premature infants) which may respond to indomethacin and small ventricular septal defects which close spontaneously. Non-structural abnormalities, e.g. polycythaemia, pulmonary hypertension, can be treated medically.

All patients with congestive cardiac failure require general measures which include administration of oxygen and diuretics, correction of acidosis, ionotropic support, restriction of fluid intake and adequate calorie intake. The only *contraindication for oxygen therapy* is the neonate in whom systemic blood flow depends on a patent ductus arteriosus (e.g. severe aortic stenosis, coarctation of the aorta, and most cases of cyanotic congenital heart disease) as it may cause ductus arteriosus closure. Such patients will benefit from prostaglandin E_1 infusion. All patients should be monitored by respiratory rate, heart size, liver size and daily weighing.

Cardiac glycosides (digoxin) are used for increasing myocardial contractility and for slowing conduction at the atrial ventricular node in paroxysmal tachycardia.

Peripheral vasodilators (captopril, nitroprusside) can be used to lower systemic vascular resistance and increase cardiac output in left ventricular output failure. All patients with uncorrected cardiac structural abnormalities require prophylaxis for subacute bacterial endocarditis. Other than in patent ductus arteriosus, secundum atrial septal defect and spontaneously closed ventricular septal defects, subacute bacterial endocarditis prophylaxis should be continued after surgical correction of structural lesions.

10 Constipation

HISTORY

By definition, constipation implies firmness or hardness of stools, rather than decreased frequency of defecation. It is therefore important to clarify this issue with the parent (or patient) when presented with this complaint. Other symptoms that may accompany constipation include abdominal pain, pain on defecation, blood streaking of stool or bleeding while passing the stool. Stool retention, either due to pain, negativism (with or without forceful toilet training), emotional problems (anxiety, depression, quiet protest or expression of anger), phobias of toilets (strange places, odours, absence of facilities or poor sanitary conditions) or postponement due to inconvenience or play may be the first trigger. Parents who train children too early or use methods that are coercive (gloved fingers, suppositories) may promote reluctance to defaecate. Chronic stool retention can present as spurious diarrhoea and/or faecal soiling. It can also present with urinary symptoms (frequency, dysuria). Certain systemic disorders such as hypothyroidism, coeliac disease, lead poisoning, neuromuscular disease and developmental handicaps can decrease gut motility and lead to stool retention. Such patients, in addition to constipation, may present with symptoms of the systemic disease.

Many formula fed infants and those that are weaned from breast milk to a milk formula may develop constipation which is mainly due to the increased protein and low carbohydrate content of the formula milk. In older children, the constipation may be due to deficient bulk.

Constipation may be a symptom in patients with intestinal obstruction but it is not the presenting complaint. Constipation may come on insidiously with malignant disease as a result of pressure on the bowel, local infiltration of bowel or impaired neurological function.

EXAMINATION

Physical examination may show features of a systemic disease such as congenital hypothyroidism (characteristic facies, protruding tongue, growth and developmental retardation), neuromuscular disease or developmental retardation. Abdominal examination may show a lump in the left lower quadrant which can be indented. The anus may show a fissure or it may be anteriorly displaced. The presence of the anal reflex indicates intact sacral function. Rectal examination allows detection of anal stricture, anal sphincter tone and contents of the rectum. In Hirschsprung's disease, the rectum is empty and constricted whereas it is dilated and filled with hard stools with chronic retention of stool (idiopathic megacolon).

MANAGEMENT

Constipation due to cow's milk formulas usually responds quickly to simple changes in either concentration of the formula, addition of some form of extra sugars (maltose, lactose or even sucrose), or fruit juices. Extra fluid intake is also helpful.

In the older child, modification of the diet may be helpful in some cases. However, in the majority of cases, constipation is due to stool retention, the cause of which has to be identified and rectified if possible. The aim of treatment in an established case of chronic constipation (reservoir syndrome) is to completely empty the bowel and to keep it emptied. This will require stool softening agents from above, such as liquid paraffin or an osmotic agent such as lactulose. These agents will soften the new stool but will have no impact on the old retained stool, though in mild cases, the new soft stool may help to "blast out" the retained stool. In severe cases, mineral oil enemas are usually needed initially to remove impacted stool. Thereafter, small enemas (twice daily in severe cases) are necessary to empty the rectum completely. This is followed by increasing doses of liquid paraffin aiming for a soft stool every day or at least every other day; if necessary with further enemas until the appropriate dose is determined. Once an appropriate dose of oil is found, that dose is maintained for many months until the bowel is allowed sufficient time to return to normal neurological function. The medication can then be gradually weaned and used in the future in short courses as necessary. General measures include good nutrition, high fibre intake and ample amounts of fluid intake.

The treatment of systemic conditions will depend on aetiology. Hirschsprung's disease has to be treated surgically.

11 Recurrent or Persistent Cough

Coughing is a reflex response to stimulation of irritant or cough receptors which are located mainly in the lower respiratory tract but are also found in the pharynx, stomach and external auditory canal. Therefore the source of a persistent cough may need to be sought beyond the respiratory tract.

HISTORY

The type of cough can aid in establishing the origin of the cough. Loose productive cough occurs in bronchitis, asthma, cystic fibrosis and bronchiectasis, brassy cough occurs in tracheitis and is also a feature of "habit cough"; croupy cough occurs in laryngitis, paroxysmal cough with or without gagging and vomiting is a feature of pertussis syndrome, foreign body and cystic fibrosis; nocturnal cough occurs in patients with hyper-reactive airways, including asthma, allergic rhinitis and sinusitis; cough which is more severe on awakening in the morning is seen in patients with cystic fibrosis, bronchiectasis, chronic bronchitis, and with post-nasal drip; cough following vigorous exercise occurs in exercise induced asthma, cystic fibrosis and bronchiectasis; and a cough that disappears with sleep is a feature of "habit cough". Additional information which may aid in the diagnosis include a history of atopy in the patient or the family which suggests an allergic aetiology; symptoms of malabsorption or family history of malabsorption indicate cystic fibrosis; symptoms related to feeding suggest aspiration; a past history of a choking episode suggests foreign body aspiration; and a smoking history in older children and adolescents suggests local irritation. A recent onset of cough associated with dyspnoea and wheezing may be due to a mediastinal mass.

EXAMINATION

This should aim to confirm the diagnosis suspected from the history. The presence of posterior nasal discharge coupled with a night cough suggests chronic upper airway disease. Atopic children may show clear mucoid discharge from the nose and have pale hypertrophied nasal mucosa. They may also show evidence of skin atopy (coarse skin or eczema). Clubbing of the digits is seen in patients with suppurative lung disease (bronchiectasis, lung abscess) but rarely in other respiratory conditions with chronic cough. Tracheal deviation is due to a shift of the mediastinum which occurs in foreign body aspiration or with a mediastinal mass.

While taking the history, the child's coughing pattern should be observed. Children who fail to cough during the consultation may do so if asked to breathe rapidly and forcefully which usually induces a cough reflex. Children with habit (tic) cough do so several times a minute with regularity.

The main aim of the chest examination is to seek for evidence of hyperinflation (loss of liver and cardiac dullness). Patients with asthma will demonstrate expiratory rhonchi which are easier to hear during forced expiration or after exercise. Coarse crepitations are heard in patients with bronchiectasis and cystic fibrosis, though they may sometimes be present in patients with acute exacerbation of asthma.

DIAGNOSIS

Sputum (if available) should be inspected and sent for microscopy and culture. The presence of eosinophils suggests asthma, while neutrophils suggest infection.

In all patients with chronic cough, a full blood count, sweat test and chest X-ray should be carried out. Patients with pulmonary haemosiderosis will have anaemia and pulmonary infiltrates, those with asthma may demonstrate eosinophilia and those with immune disorders may demonstrate deficiency of neutrophils or lymphocytes. An infiltrate on chest X-ray may establish a diagnosis or indicate that further investigations are required, e.g. tuberclin test for hilar lymph node enlargement, screening for suspected foreign body aspiration. Further investigations such as X-ray of the paranasal sinuses, barium swallow, special bacteriological studies, bronchoscopy and evaluation of ciliary morphology or function will depend on the initial evaluation.

12 Crying Babies

Parents frequently seek help for crying babies. This may be partly due to society's expectation that babies should not cry if they are fed, changed and kept warm. Parents may believe that the baby is in pain, and wonder whether an underlying disease needs to be treated.

HISTORY

The history should be taken in a relaxed and unhurried atmosphere. If a baby cries inconsolably, it may be preferable for someone else to look after the infant during the interview. However, most mothers will not be able to relax if they can hear their baby crying in a stranger's arms or if they are dissuaded from going to their baby's aid. The parents may already have a theory for the cause of crying. It is important to let them talk about it and describe the strategies that they have already tried. More information should be obtained about the crying: when it occurs, is there periodicity, is there any pattern, is there any relief with medications, rocking or when walking or when travelling in the car or something else? At what age did it start? The feeding history should include information on sucking pattern of the infant, frequency of feeds, vomiting after feeds and whether the baby is happy after feeding. The baby's sleeping pattern and weight gain should be noted. The stool consistency and frequency should be recorded.

In all crying babies, the social history is very important. The parents' support system, expectations and environmental stress factor should be elucidated. These may include lack of sleep, demands of other siblings, post-natal depression or anxiety, an unhelpful spouse or interference by mother or mother-in-law — all of which may interfere with the parents' ability to rear the child. Any of these factors may be compounded by the unhelpful advice offered by well-meaning friends, relatives and health professionals.

PHYSICAL EXAMINATION

Usually no abnormalities are found. In underfed babies, the weight gain is poor (less than 100g/week) and they may show a drop in the centiles. Over-stimulated babies are tense and avoid eye contact with the examiner. In babies with frequent stools due to lactose intolerance, a nappy rash may be present. Besides a general physical examination, special attention should be paid to the examination of the nervous system to exclude a neurological abnormality and examination of the abdomen to exclude an acute abdomen. The baby should be observed while feeding and a note should be made of mother and baby interaction. It should be remembered that any judgement about the parent/child interaction is made under adverse conditions and over a very brief period. Such judgements influence the tone of the examination and, if negative, can easily undermine parents' confidence.

MANAGEMENT

Treatment of crying babies is difficult. The most important first step is to ensure (from the history and the physical examination) that there is no underlying disease process such as underfeeding (poor weight gain), gastro-oesophageal reflux manifested as recurrent vomiting and restlessness after vomiting, over-stimulation, an acute abdomen (obstructed hernias, definite guarding and area of tenderness) and lactose intolerance — manifested by rapid weight gain, frequent loose stools, nappy rash and more than 0.5% reducing substances in the stools. Urinary tract infection may present as crying but is difficult to exclude without urine examination.

In the majority of cases, no physical cause will be found. It is important to reassure the parents of such babies that there is no reason to suspect that the baby is in pain. This does not mean that there is no underlying physical cause (maybe the physician is not sufficiently clever to detect it!) or that there is nothing wrong with the baby. There obviously is, but the reason is obscure and may never be known. To dismiss crying as "behavioural" is unhelpful, states the obvious and conveys to many parents that the fault is all theirs. Whether the baby is in pain, distress or discomfort, the baby needs the comfort *and the parents need permission to give it* — that would be the most helpful thing the doctor could do in many cases.

Some parents need support and understanding in order to help them to cope with the problem. Many parents are worried that they may spoil the baby if picked up and comforted when crying or that the baby may suffer psychological damage if not picked up immediately the crying starts. These issues need to be discussed in the light of the infant's cognitive and emotional stage of development and *without resorting to advice which is based on popular but unsubstantiated beliefs.* Some mothers may need more direction than others, for example, about regular schedules for feeding and naps, whereas others may need to be encouraged to be less rigid about these kinds of things. Very active babies may need more help to calm down than those that are more placid by nature. The adverse environmental factors which may be compounding the problem need to be taken into account. Most of these, for example, an unhelpful spouse or a neighbour who hammers on the walls, will not be able to be readily changed but strategies can be discussed for coping with them. Depressed mothers may need psychiatric help. Specific treatment may be needed for those infants with physical problems such as gastro-oesophageal reflux.

Medications are rarely useful in the management of crying babies partly because most parents believe it is wrong and even harmful to use them. Those that have been used include anti-histamines, anti-spasmodics and hypnotics.

13 Depression in Childhood

Disorders of affect can occur in children of any age including early infancy. Transient periods of depressed mood and diminished pleasure in usual activities are frequent among children and adolescents. In true depression, these periods are persistent for weeks. These symptoms may be "masked" with additional symptoms of other conditions such as hyperactivity, learning disabilities, enuresis and encopresis. The history should be obtained from multiple sources: the child, the parents, the school and other concerned adults (e.g. grandparents).

HISTORY

Depression in *early infancy* is classically seen in disrupted mother/child relationships. In extreme cases, death may occur. Common presentations include failure to thrive and delay in motor, social and language development. By six months of age, infants respond to separation first by protest followed by apathy and sad facial expression. Affected infants cry silently and stare into space.

In *children* symptoms vary according to age. Younger children express feelings non-verbally and in play activities, while older children are able to describe their symptoms and often give a more accurate account of their fantasies and thoughts than adults.

Symptoms occur in the following domains:

1. mood: sad, low, unhappy, empty, bad, easy tears, irritability
2. behaviour: social withdrawal and loss of interests in usual activities, loss of pleasure (anhedonia) in such things as friendships, sports, games and family outings; depending on personality, the child may

become clinging and dependent; aloof, withdrawn and seclusive; or more destructive, aggressive and defiant
3. vegetative: sleep and appetite disturbance, apathy, poor concentration
4. talk: feeling hopeless and helpless; being ugly, stupid, worthless and unloved; suicidal preoccupations
5. thoughts and play: themes of mistreatment, loss and abandonment, being criticised and blamed; injury, death and suicide

Hyperactivity, aggression, conduct symptoms, somatic symptoms (stomachaches, headaches) and drug and alcohol abuse (in adolescents) may co-occur with these symptoms, but only mask them in so far as the diagnosis of depression is not considered.

There may be particular stressor(s) associated with the onset of the depression, e.g. a loss or an interpersonal conflict. A family history of psychiatric disorder is often present, and one or both parents may be depressed; there may also be a background of discord, abuse or neglect.

It is important to have a reasonable index of suspicion and to be willing to ask about suicidal ideation and behaviour; broaching the topic is far better than not doing so and adolescents if asked will generally admit to current ideation, past attempts and exposure to suicide.

EXAMINATION

Clinically depressed children often look sad and depressed, are tearful, have slow movements and may speak in a hopeless and despairing manner.

Parents may be noted to be anxious or depressed.

MANAGEMENT

Assessment of the likelihood of suicide and need for safety is the first priority. This requires assessing whether the family is able to keep the child or adolescent safe, and providing alternative short-term care if this is not possible, e.g. hospitalisation after a suicide attempt.

The value of using antidepressants in prepubertal depression has not been conclusively established. If they are to be used, adequate precautions especially in relation to cardiotoxity should be taken, because of a small number of sudden deaths that have occurred in children on tricyclic antidepressants. Parental and family assessment and therapy is a mainstay of treatment at all ages, where the family is intact, or if this is not the case, with the child's caregivers/guardians. Cognitive behavioural therapy, individual psychotherapy, and groups aiming at social skills training and self-esteem building may be indicated with older children and adolescents.

14 Developmental Delay

Developmental disability is relatively common occurring at a rate of 7–9 per 1000 live births.

PRESENTATION AND HISTORY

A developmental problem can present in a number of ways:

1. A condition known to be associated with developmental disability may be evident at or soon after birth, e.g. Down syndrome (Fig. 14.1).
2. Delay may be detected on routine screening especially at the Early Childhood Centres.
3. The parents may express concern that the child is not achieving important milestones, especially walking or speech, as quickly as other children of the same age.
4. Other agencies, particularly preschool or school, may see that the child is "different" from peers and lacks skills appropriate for his/her age.
5. More subtle signs: especially in infancy, neurodevelopmental problems may first make their presence known through more subtle and general concerns. The most frequent are feeding problems. In full term babies, persisting problems such as poor sucking, lack of interest in feeds or very slow feeding are unusual after the first week or so and if such problems continue when there is no reason (such as urinary tract infection or other medical conditions) one should consider the possibility of a neurodevelopmental disorder and at least follow the baby's development closely.

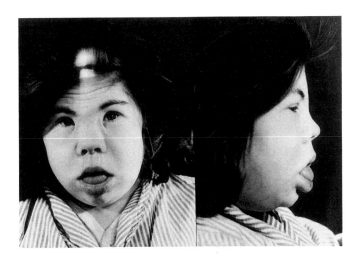

Fig. 14.1 *Down syndrome.* Note typical facies with epicanthic folds, flat nasal bridge and large tongue.

In the pregnancy and birth history, one should inquire about illnesses (especially febrile episodes) and ingestion of drugs including tobacco and alcohol. Details of labour and delivery and the baby's condition at birth should be sought. These include birth weight (was it similar to other siblings), Apgar scores, difficulties in establishing respiration, hypoglycaemia, hyperbilirubinaemia and feeding difficulties.

A history of behaviour in infancy may provide suggestive evidence of a developmental problem which existed from early infancy: was the baby excessively irritable, perhaps resisting cuddling? On the other hand, the child may have been unusually "good", sleeping more than other babies of the same age and taking little interest in the surroundings. The mother may have noticed that the baby "felt different" to her previous children, being either more stiff or more floppy or limp than usual. In addition to a standard medical history, the doctor should ask specifically about the child's developmental milestones (Table 14.1). An important question is whether the child has actually lost skills that were present before. This may lead to the first suspicion of a neurodegenerative disorder.

A detailed family history is important. One should inquire about consanguinity of parents, miscarriages and similar illnesses in siblings

Table 14.1 Major Developmental Milestones

1. MOTOR MILESTONES

	Average	Upper Limit of Normal
Lifts head in prone	6 weeks	8 weeks
Head control on pull-to-sit	3 months	4 months
Rolls over	5 months	6 months
Sits without support	7 months	8 months
Crawls on hands and knees	9 months	10 months
Pulls to stand on furniture	10 months	11 months
Walks with one hand held	11 months	12 months
Walks independently	13 months	16 months
Runs	18 months	21 months
Jumps off floor	21 months	24 months
Jumps off step	25 months	28 months
Pedals tricycle	36 months	42 months

2. SPEECH AND LANGUAGE MILESTONES

"Coos" in social response	6 weeks	8 weeks
Laughs aloud	3 months	4 months
Babbles	6 months	7 months
Double syllables (da-da,ba-ba)	7 months	9 months
Strings of syllables (da-da-da-da)	9 months	10 months
Waves bye-bye	9 months	12 months
Meaningful words (3)	12 months	14 months
Vocabulary of 10 + words	18 months	21 months
Spontaneously names common objects as he/she encounters them	21 months	24 months
Two word combinations	21 months	24 months
Names pictures of familiar items	21 months	24 months
Three-four word sentences	24 months	30 months
Complex sentences (two verbs)	36 months	42 months
Asks where and when questions	36 months	42 months
Asks why questions	42 months	48 months

Can narrate events, a story etc in well formed sentences with reasonable sequence	48 months	54 months

3. COGNITIVE SKILLS

(a) **Block Play**	**Average**	**Upper Limit of Normal**
Two block tower	13 months	16 months
Three block tower	15 months	18 months
Spontaneous container play: puts blocks and other items in and out of container	18 months	21 months
Four-six block tower	24 months	30 months
Train of blocks	24 months	30 months
Bridge of three blocks	36 months	42 months
Elaborate, imaginative constructions	48 months	

(b) PENCIL AND PAPER SKILLS

Makes random marks on paper	13 months	15 months
Spontaneous to-and-fro scribble	16 months	24 months
Circular scribble	21 months	24 months
Imitates horizontal and vertical lines	24 months	30 months
Makes "spiral" in attempting to copy circle	33 months	36 months
Copies circle correctly	36 months	42 months

and close relatives. One should also inquire about the school progress of the parents and their siblings; about relatives in previous generations who may have been in residential institutions or who had seizures or who were late in walking or talking. Ask whom in the family the child "takes after" in looks and temperament: this may provide a clue to a possible dysmorphic syndrome.

EXAMINATION

The examination of a baby or young child suspected of developmental delay begins with observation of general demeanour and play during the history taking session. Offer the child a few everyday toys. Note the quality and spontaneity of the child's engagement with his/her family members and with the doctor. Observe how he or she manipulates and uses the toys: does he/she explore the attributes and detail of the toys? Does he/she relate two or more objects meaningfully, e.g. putting a spoon in a cup, making a tower of blocks or putting objects in and out of a small container? The child with a developmental disability may demonstrate a restricted and non-functional type of play, e.g. repetitively casting or mouthing objects or becoming obsessed with spinning the wheels of a small car.

If possible, observe the child when he/she is placed on the floor. How does he/she move about? Does he/she move easily in and out of different positions such as supine to sitting, crawling to sitting, standing and walking? There may be unusual patterns of movement such as kicking along on his back which raises the suspicion of cerebral palsy.

On physical examination there may be some indications of underlying cause of the child's developmental delay. Height, weight and head circumference are important measurements: marked variation from what is normal for age and the family pattern may be due to prenatal infection or to a congenital anomaly syndrome. The child may give a general impression of unusual appearance and detailed examination may confirm the presence of three or more dysmorphic features.

A careful examination of the skin may reveal the presence of lesions associated with the neurocutaneous syndromes, especially the cafe-au-lait patches suggestive of neurofibromatosis or the white ovoid spots of tuberous sclerosis (Fig. 14.2). These latter are best seen under a Wood's light: in the absence of this, a small hand held ultra-violet torch is helpful in a darkened room.

Neurological examination may reveal alterations in muscle tone: mild diffuse hypotonia is not an uncommon association with general developmental delay but may be due to neuromuscular disorders, cerebellar disorders or the low-tone forms of cerebral palsy. Hypertonia, a recognised feature of cerebral palsy, may not be evident until after the first year of life. The diagnosis may be suspected in early infancy by the

This complex set of actions should commence with referral to a paediatrician who arranges and coordinates the further referrals. The assessment process involves the cooperation of paediatrician with psychologist, social worker and other professionals, e.g. occupational therapist, physiotherapist and speech pathologist in a coordinated team approach.

Intervention programmes also involve an interdisciplinary approach with contributions from special education teachers, therapists and various community resources such as pre-schools.

Medical investigation into aetiology is guided by the clinical picture: there is no list of "routine" tests to be carried out in every case of developmental disability. However virtually every child with developmental delay should have a chromosome study carried out, including a search for the fragile X site (FraXq27) which must be requested specifically as the cells require a different culture medium.

Other common tests include a urinary metabolic screen to exclude relatively common metabolic disorders (if a rarer condition is suspected on clinical grounds, e.g. mucopolysaccharide disorder, a specific request is made).

A CAT or MRI scan is indicated where developmental delay is associated with neurological signs or a seizure disorder and if a neurocutaneous or neurodegenerative disorder is suspected. In other cases, the likely yield of information should be balanced against the possible hazards (in most cases small) of anaesthesia which is usually required for very young children.

In boys with developmental delay, especially if associated with any degree of hypotonia, a serum creatine phosphokinase is necessary to exclude Duchenne muscular dystrophy which sometimes presents with mild general delay before the motor deterioration becomes evident. As this condition carries a high risk of recurrence within the family, early diagnosis of the index case is important.

Other tests are indicated on clinical grounds, e.g. tests for prenatal infection, for hypothyroidism, calcium and phosphate disturbance, and skeletal radiological studies.

All children with developmental delay should have formal audiometry testing and an ophthalmological examination to exclude hearing and vision impairment as a causative or complicating factor in their delay.

Any child in whom there is a suspicion of loss of previously acquired skills should be referred to a paediatric neurologist for further investigation such as lysozomal enzymes, lactate/pyruvate studies, and rectal biopsy. Most neurodegenerative disorders are genetic and carry a high recurrence risk.

15 Acute Diarrhoea with Vomiting

In an average year, the World Health Organisation reckons there are 3 to 5 billion episodes of acute diarrhoea worldwide and on average 5 to 10 million deaths in childhood. While most of these deaths occur in infancy and malnutrition plays a large role, deaths also occur due to inappropriate treatment or undertreatment of fluid and electrolyte disturbances. Infants particularly are at risk of dying due to acute gastroenteritis for two reasons: they have a higher proportion of extracellular fluid volume which is available for exchange across the gut mucosa and they have a huge gut mucosal surface relative to their size. Acute gastroenteritis is usually caused by viruses and has its peak in the winter months whereas bacterial infections occur all year round with a slight preponderance during the summer months.

HISTORY

The presenting symptom is frequent fluid stools and increased volume of faeces. The stools rarely contain blood or mucus. Vomiting may or may not be present. Respiratory symptoms such as cough and rhinorrhoea may precede the gastrointestinal symptoms and fever and mild abdominal pain may also be present. About 40% of infants with Rotavirus gastroenteritis will have some mild respiratory symptoms and children with bacterial gastroenteritis tend to have higher fevers and more abdominal pain and toxicity. In infants who are dehydrated, urine output will be diminished. Previous growth parameters will indicate whether the child is thriving.

EXAMINATION

The degree of dehydration is the first and the most important thing to assess. Very mild dehydration (less than 5%) shows an alert infant who may be thirsty, a little restless and passing concentrated urine of smaller volume infrequently. Moderate dehydration (5–10%) causes increasing thirst and restlessness, irritability and some lethargy, a rising pulse rate, normal blood pressure, sunken eyes and, in infancy sunken anterior fontanelle together with some loss of skin elasticity which may take between 1 and 2 second to bounce back after pinching.

Severe dehydration (greater than 10%) results in infants appearing drowsy, limp, cold, sweaty, cyanosed and drowsy with gradual progression to coma. Older children become apprehensive, cold, sweaty and eventually cyanosed. The pulse rate increases and the blood pressure starts to fall, the eyes are sunken as is the fontanelle and skin elasticity takes more than 2 seconds to return after pinching. Anuria occurs with this degree of dehydration.

Abdominal tenderness is absent in viral gastroenteritis, but may be present to a mild degree with bacterial infections. There are no masses and the rest of the examination is unremarkable. The infant's weight and height should be recorded.

DIAGNOSIS

Not all acute vomiting and diarrhoea is due to gastroenteritis and particularly so if the vomitus contains bile or blood, if there is severe abdominal pain, and if there is severe toxaemia or fever, abdominal distension, tenderness, guarding or an abdominal mass. As neonates may be suffering from Hirschsprung's enterocolitis or necrotising enterocolitis, the diagnosis should not be accepted without caution. Failure to thrive prior to the onset of acute vomiting and diarrhoea is another warning signal that there may be other underlying problems.

Urinary tract infection, pneumonia and occasionally septicaemia may also mimic gastroenteritis. Surgical conditions including appendicitis, intussusception, partial bowel obstruction and Hirschsprung's disease must be considered in atypical cases. Rarer causes include diabetes mellitis, antibiotic diarrhoea and haemolytic-uraemic syndrome.

In acute vomiting and diarrhoea the commonest single cause is Rotavirus gastroenteritis and other viruses. Bacteria such as campylobacter, salmonella and shigella account for typically less than 10% of acute illnesses, and protozoa such as giardia and amoebae are very uncommon causes of acute vomiting and diarrhoea in infancy and childhood.

MANAGEMENT

Ideally, urinalysis should be performed on any child appearing to have acute gastroenteritis. Stool microscopy and culture is particularly appropriate when there is a good deal of pain associated with diarrhoea, when there is blood in the stool, if diarrhoea persists for more than a week, when there has been recent overseas travel, when an epidemic is suspected or if the child is in an institution. In general, if the child is not sick enough to be in hospital, he does not warrant blood counts or serum electrolytes.

There are essentially 2 aims in the treatment of acute vomiting and diarrhoea, namely, the restoration and maintenance of fluid and electrolyte balance and the restoration rapidly of normal nutrition.

Antibiotics, anti-emetics and anti-diarrhoea agents play a minor role in the management of such infants and young children. Treatment of shigella (with ampicillan, co-trimoxazole or chloramphenicol) and campylobacter (with erythromycin) is reasonable if the child's symptoms are continuing significantly when the culture report comes through. As campylobacter can occasionally cause a relapse in illness, it may also be reasonable to treat if it relapses. Otherwise antibiotics should not be used.

Anti-emetics are neither necessary nor indicated in acute gastroenteritis. There is a significant risk of dystonic reactions as well.

Anti-diarrhoea agents, because they do not address the basic pathophysiology of fluid loss from the gut mucosa, are useless and sometimes dangerous in infants and young children.

Fluid and electrolyte therapy is the mainstay of treatment. Infants and children, who are either not dehydrated or only very mildly dehydrated, usually only require 24 to 48 hours of dietary modification. If an infant is breastfed, in general such an infant may continue to be breastfed although extra water for fluid losses may be required. In bottle-fed babies, milk formula as well as solids should be ceased for about 24 hours and replaced with clear fluids. Solids may be reintroduced in 24 to 48 hours even if there is persistent diarrhoea. Clear fluids may include cordial, lemonade, fruit juice or fruit juice drinks but they must be diluted, cordial 1 in 6 with water, the others 1 in 4 with water. If vomiting is a major feature, acidic fruit juices should be avoided. Glucose powder (Glucodin) 1 teaspoon per 120 mls is also appropriate but in general, oral rehydration solutions* such as Gastrolyte are unnecessary in non-dehydrated infants and children. Oral rehydrating solutions are very acceptable in mild, moderate and even severe dehydration, but there is a very small risk of over dependence on this agent and there is also the risk of inappropriate dilution (in water) creating electrolyte disturbances.

It is quite reasonable to treat an infant or young child at home with mild gastroenteritis providing the family is able to cope and the infant's fluid intake is appropriate without excessive persistent vomiting and that other diagnoses are unlikely. However, if the infant fails to improve, if the diagnosis is in doubt, if the infant is under 6 months of age, or if there is pre-existing disease particularly cardiac or renal, the infant should be referred to hospital. However, if the family is unable to cope or if an infant is dehydrated or has persistent vomiting, such infants generally need admission to hospital.

---

*An appropriate home-made oral rehydrating fluid could be made by adding 4 tablespoons of cane sugar, 1/2 teaspoonful of salt to a litre of water and bringing the solution to the boil.

16 Chronic Diarrhoea

HISTORY

When presented with a child with chronic diarrhoea, the physician must decide whether the stool pattern is abnormal, e.g. normal breastfed infants may have 6–8 loose stools a day. It is also important to distinguish between watery and loose stools as the latter may be normal.

In the newborn period, persistent diarrhoea may be a symptom of drug withdrawal or Hirschsprung's disease — the latter will give a history of a delay in passage of meconium or constipation prior to the onset of diarrhoea. Between the age of 6 months to 3 years, many children have intermittent loose stools with no apparent cause (toddler's diarrhoea). The stools occur early in the day and not during the night. The infants appear healthy and are gaining weight satisfactorily. The stools are loose but not watery. They usually occur immediately after a feed and contain peas and carrots and tend to be offensive in odour.

In all children with chronic diarrhoea a dietary history must be obtained. In some cases the parents may already have observed the association of diarrhoea with the consumption of certain foods, e.g. fructose, sucrose. In other cases, it may not be so obvious as in a child who may be consuming large quantities of fruit juices, cordials containing sorbitol or in secondary lactose intolerance following an acute attack of diarrhoea. The presence of blood in the stool should alert the physician to the possibility of food intolerance including cow's milk allergy which may occur even in breastfed infants. Most frequently the blood in the stool may be a symptom of infection such as Yersinia, Campylobacter, Salmonella, Shigella or Giardia *lamblia* (Fig. 16.1). Blood and mucus in the stool also may be the presenting symptom of ulcerative colitis or Crohn's disease.

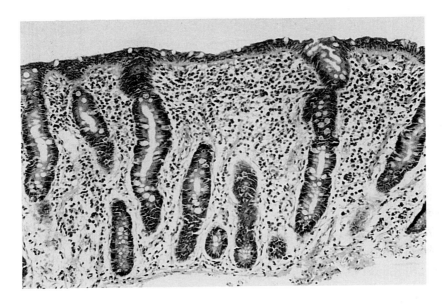

Fig. 16.1 *Giardia lamblia* seen in small intestine biopsy.

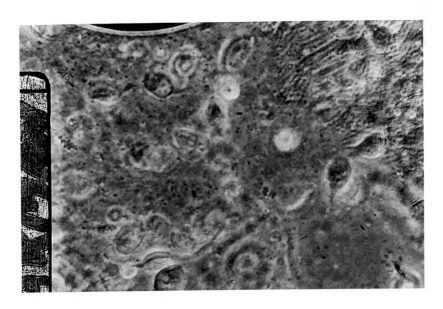

Fig. 16.2 *Coeliac disease.* Small intestine biopsy shows complete villus atrophy, large crypts and infiltration with round cells.

Additional symptoms in infants and children with malabsorption syndromes which typically cause diarrhoea are large foul smelling stools and growth failure. The symptoms may be present from birth in cystic fibrosis or may occur a few months after the introduction of gluten containing foods (wheat, oats, barley and rye) in coeliac disease (Fig. 16.2). Whereas the infant with cystic fibrosis may have respiratory symptoms and have a voracious appetite, those with coeliac disease are irritable and have poor appetite and recurrent vomiting.

Diarrhoea may be the presenting symptom in infants with many systemic diseases, though such patients may also have other symptoms which may give a clue to the diagnosis. Patients with intestinal lymphangiectasis may have peripheral oedema and recurrent infections. Those with acrodermatitis enteropathica have a typical skin rash involving the perianal and perioral regions. Patients with immune disorders present with recurrent infections and those with hormone related diarrhoea may present with a mass in the abdomen due to a neural crest tumour.

All the conditions causing diarrhoea in infancy and early childhood can cause diarrhoea in older children. The other conditions that need to be considered in the differential diagnosis are irritable bowel which presents with recurrent cramping abdominal pain and stools which may alternate from diarrhoea to constipation. Inflammatory bowel disease in this age group has a variable presentation and may present besides diarrhoea with systemic evidence of inflammation (fever, weight loss), abdominal pain, blood in the stool, perianal disease (Fig. 16.3), anaemia or extra-intestinal manifestations (arthralgia, arthritis and erythema nodosum). In such patients, growth failure can occur or precede the other symptoms.

Occasionally chronic constipation with overflow incontinence will manifest as diarrhoea. The history will reveal that the problem began with constipation.

EXAMINATION

The aim of the examination is to determine whether the child is sick or well, whether he is thriving or not, whether there are signs of anaemia,

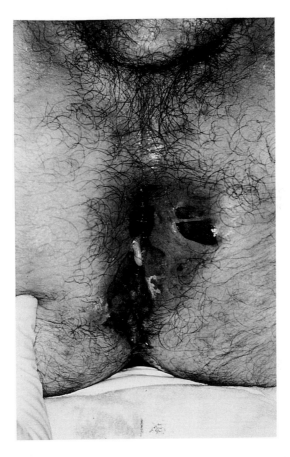

Fig. 16.3 Anal fissures and fistulae in a child with *Crohn's disease.*

abdominal tenderness or masses. The physician should look for evidence of other physical signs which indicate a systemic disease and the cause of the diarrhoea.

MANAGEMENT

In all cases stool microscopy and culture should be carried out. The aim of the microscopy examination is to look for blood, white blood cells, ova, cysts (giardia, Entamoeba histolytica), parasites, fat globules and fatty acid crystals. The stools should also be tested for reducing substances. Urine analysis should be carried out in all patients as chronic diarrhoea may be the presenting symptom of urinary tract infection. Further investigations will depend on whether the problem is perceived to be a small bowel, large bowel or a systemic disease.

Simple dietary measures may be adequate in the majority of patients with chronic diarrhoea who have food intolerances or are consuming large quantities of carbohydrates. In infants with persistent diarrhoea after an acute episode, restriction of lactose for a short period will alleviate the problem. Treatment for children with toddler's diarrhoea may include restricting the frequency of feeding, restricting the volume of fluids ingested, avoiding excessive intake of juices and reassuring the parents. A high fat diet may be helpful in some children. A therapeutic trial with metronidazole (Flagyl) may be useful in some cases of undiagnosed chronic diarrhoea even though there may be no cysts or parasites demonstrated on stool examination.

17 The Dysmorphic Child

HISTORY

The dysmorphic features may be noted by the physician on routine examination of the child or it may be a concern expressed by a nurse or the parents. They may also be observed when examining an unexplained stillborn baby. In most cases the problem is recognised at or soon after birth; in some cases the infant is seen because of feeding problems, failing to thrive or developmental retardation. The parents may not express their concern as they fear the worst and it may be necessary to prompt them to ask questions. In all cases, the physician should inquire whether the child resembles any other member of the family. Besides the family history, the physician should inquire about maternal age and previous pregnancies, maternal past and present illnesses, maternal health (infections) and drug intake during pregnancy, foetal activity *in utero*, gestational age, the baby's weight, height and head circumference at birth, baby's immediate problems after birth and the baby's subsequent growth and development. The history will aid the physician to establish an aetiological diagnosis and to determine whether the baby was small for dates and developing normally.

EXAMINATION

The word dysmorphic is a "first glance" diagnosis. The next step is to analyse what component of the baby's features makes one think that the baby looks unusual and see whether it can be backed-up with some concrete minor congenital abnormality. These include abnormalities of the cranium (abnormal shape, sutures and fontanelle), eyes (widely

spaced, epicanthic folds, Brushfield spots), mouth (too large tongue for
mouth, or too small mouth for tongue, cleft palate, micrognathia), ears
(low set, abnormal configuration), hands and feet (broad and short,
Simian crease, abnormal dermatoglyphics, clinodactyly, broad thumb
nails, nail hypoplasia, talipes), extra digits (Fig. 17.1), joints
(contractures or decreased mobility), skin (deep pigmented patches or
lines of deep pigmentation, small patches of aplasia of the skin on the
scalp, excessive skin folds at the back of the neck, excessive hairiness),
genitalia (hypospadias, cryptorchidism) and muscle tone. The initial
conclusion should be confirmed by measurement for comparison with
normals for weight, height, head circumference, chest, hand, feet, outer-
canthal distance, inner-canthal distance, inter-pupillary distance and
palpebral length, fontanelle, ear length, penile length and growth and
testicular growth.

A thorough physical examination should be performed to determine
if there are associated somatic abnormalities. Hearing and vision should
be evaluated and fundoscopic examination carried out. In addition to
the physical examination, a developmental assessment should be carried
out in all patients.

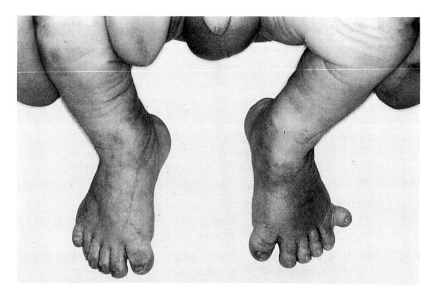

Fig. 17.1 Six toes in an infant with *Ellis-van Creveld syndrome.*

MANAGEMENT

If the baby is stillborn, in order to make a definite diagnosis, physical abnormalities should be recorded in detail. In addition, the baby should be photographed with a polaroid camera and have a skeletal survey and chromosome analysis (skin, cord, blood) carried out. Whenever possible, an autopsy should be arranged.

If the baby is a newborn of normal birth weight and there are no obvious concerns, it is necessary to decide whether the clinical findings are sufficient to warrant further investigations. It is a great help if some concrete mild congenital abnormality is present to support the clinical impression. Without strong supportive evidence, it is justified to wait a few days to see whether facial features subsequently appear more normal, as sometimes intra-uterine compression will give the clinical impression of an abnormal face. It is always important to have seen the facial configuration of both parents. Frequently it may be found that one of the parents has some of the same dysmorphic features. This can of course reflect a dominantly inherited condition but may be within the range of normal variation. In some situations it is better to defer discussion about a baby's appearance until the baby is established at home and the parents are bonded. It is always better to discuss the specific feature, e.g. "the eyes are widely set" rather than imply that the whole face is abnormal.

A correct diagnosis of a specific syndrome is necessary to provide a prognosis and plan of management for the affected infant as well as genetic counselling for parents. The prime investigation that often helps is chromosome analysis. Sometimes this is better left to be ordered by the paediatrician as the laboratory may require indications to use special techniques for diagnosis, e.g. prophase banding for Prader Willi syndrome, use of folic acid deficient media for fragile X syndrome. In at least 50% of children who look dysmorphic, no definite diagnosis is made. It is reasonable to have such children reviewed every 3–5 years by a geneticist or a paediatrician as syndrome diagnosis is a rapidly changing field with new entities being defined and diagnostic techniques being improved.

Many well recognised syndromes have a genetic basis though no specific tests are available for diagnosis. It follows that unless the diagnosis is obvious, all patients with dysmorphic features should be referred to a paediatrician or a geneticist for an opinion.

18 Dysuria

Dysuria is defined as pain or difficulty in passing urine. It rarely occurs as an isolated symptom and its aetiology is identified in most cases by considering the associated symptoms.

HISTORY

In infants, crying is the most common symptom which is associated with micturition. The crying stops with cessation of micturition. The crying is accompanied with flexion of the thighs and is often described as colic. Other symptoms include hyper-irritability and frequency of micturition manifested as frequent wet nappies.

In young children, crying with micturition is more readily identified. These patients tend to delay urination as long as possible which results in suprapubic discomfort due to bladder distention. They have a hesitant or episodic urinary stream because of difficulty in initiating or continuing urination.

Older children are able to indicate discomfort and difficulty in the act of voiding. They may use terms such as "burn", "hurt" or "it is hard to pass urine" to describe the pain.

In all age groups, it is important to inquire about perineal infections, other urinary symptoms, (such as haematuria, foul smelling urine, frequency of micturition), urethral or vaginal discharge, use of bubble baths or perfumed soaps and non-specific symptoms such as fever, malaise, loss of appetite, abdominal pain, diarrhoea or vomiting.

EXAMINATION

In all cases, the external genitalia should be examined for meatal ulceration and congenital abnormalities (hypospadias, urethral prolapse in girls). The vagina should be examined for the presence of erythema, vesicles and discharge.

The abdomen should be palpated for suprapubic and costovertebral tenderness, abdominal masses (enlarged bladder, ureters or kidneys) and evidence of constipation.

DIAGNOSIS AND MANAGEMENT

Unless the cause of dysuria is obvious, e.g. local ulceration, urinary tract infection should be sought in all patients with dysuria. Clinical impression is not sufficient for a diagnosis or exclusion of urinary tract infection. Microbiological confirmation is necessary. Diagnosis is facilitated by appropriate collection and transport of the urine to the laboratory. "Clean catch" mid stream urine collection into a sterile container which should be placed in a refrigerator at 4°C pending dispatch to the laboratory is satisfactory for less urgent cases. In the "septic" neonate or the unwell baby for whom immediate antibiotic treatment is planned after collection of specimen for laboratory evaluation, direct urine collection by bladder aspiration or failing this, catheterisation are the preferred options. Direct urine collection may also be necessary when doubtful results are received from the laboratory following urine collection by other methods. A "bag" urine is most useful if it does not show infection. If organisms are cultured in significant numbers from a "bag" collection, confirmation by more reliable methods should be instituted prior to therapy. Bacterial colony counts of 10^5 or more/ml of urine of a single organism, if confirmed, are diagnostic of urinary tract infection. 10^3 organisms per ml from a catheter specimen or ANY colony growth from a bladder aspirate are suggestive of urinary tract infection.

The finding of more than 10 white cells/ml of urine with a positive culture is helpful in diagnosis of urinary tract infection, but a normal leucocyte count in the urine does not exclude it.

Dipsticks have been used for the diagnosis of urinary tract infection but they have their limitation. Leukocytes esterase test is not specific for urine infection. The nitrite test has to be performed immediately after collection on the first urine passed in the morning, but it is negative in infections due to pseudomonas or streptococci as neither of these organisms convert nitrate to nitrite. A positive Albustix *does not* indicate urinary tract infection.

An outline of the management of a patient with proven urinary tract infection is shown in Fig. 18.1. Figure 18.2 shows a micturating cystourethrogram taken of an infant with severe vesicoureteric reflux.

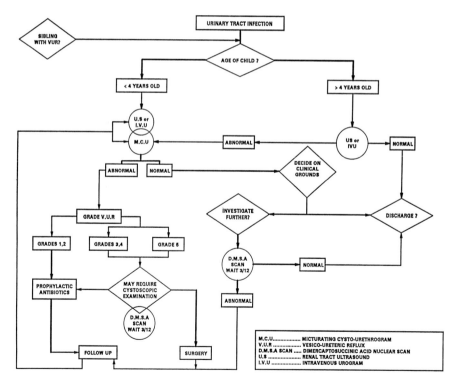

Fig. 18.1   Investigation of childhood urinary tract infection.

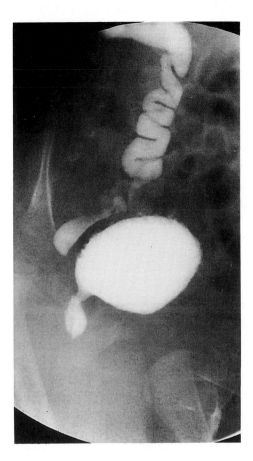

Fig. 18.2 Micturating cystourethrogram shows severe *vesicoureteric reflux* in an infant with urinary tract infection.

19 Middle Ear Infection

Inflammation of the middle ear is a common disease of childhood and requires early and adequate treatment to avoid complications.

HISTORY

In acute otitis media the symptoms are fever, pain in the ear and hearing loss. In the *infant*, the pain in the ear may be manifested as irritability, crying and pulling on the ear. Hearing loss may be overlooked. In *older children*, the hearing loss may be obvious or the parents may complain of the child being inattentive or there may be disturbance of speech. Otitis media with perforation may present as earaches or as a persistent discharge.

EXAMINATION

In otitis externa, there may be excoriation of the auditory canal. In some cases a furuncle is present. These patients are afebrile. Tenderness is often elicited by gently pulling on the ear lobe.

In acute otitis media, the eardrum is hyperaemic, opaque, bulging and demonstrates poor mobility. Purulent material may be seen in the auditory canal. The fever may be high and the patient appears toxic and may be in distress.

In children with chronic otitis media, the tympanic membrane is either retracted or convex. It is usually opaque and demonstrates poor mobility. Fluid may be observed behind the ear drum. Hearing loss may be demonstrated clinically or by audiometry which shows conduction hearing loss.

MANAGEMENT

Acute otitis media is usually treated as a bacterial infection in spite of many cases being viral in origin. Common organisms that have been isolated include *Strep. pneumoniae, H. influenzae* and *Strep. pyogenes.* Amoxycillin which is effective against all these three organisms is the antibiotic of choice.

Supportive therapy includes analgesics and antipyretics. Oral and topical nasal decongestants may be helpful.

Otitis media with effusion requires no treatment in most cases. However if hearing loss is severe, persistent and affects language development, a trial of antibiotics and nasal decongestants may be effective. If these measures fail, inserting a ventilation or tympanostomy (grommet) tube is indicated.

20 Eating Problems

Eating problems are among the commonest problems with infants, children and adolescents. The presentation will vary with age. Changes in weight require medical intervention.

HISTORY

A. *Early infancy (birth to 6 months)*: The physician should determine the exact nature of the feeding problems which may include difficulty in attachment at the breast, difficulty in sucking, crying during feeds, vomiting or being unsettled between feeds (see Breastfeeding Problems, Crying Babies, Recurrent Vomiting). Tiredness during feeds suggests a cardiorespiratory problem. Irritability may be due to a neurological problem or the temperament of the infant. A variety of parental problems may be noted: maternal isolation, paternal unavailability, marital problems, psychiatric disorders including post-natal depression and anxiety, alcoholism and also poverty and social disadvantage. Feeding situations may be unsatisfying and non-feeding interactions difficult or impoverished. Child abuse and domestic violence may be contributing to the problem. In some infants, physical interventions in the neonatal period such as insertion of a naso-gastric tube, parenteral feeding or the creation of a gastrostomy may have impaired the acquisition of normal feeding skills.

B. *6–15 months*: The major problem in this age group is the issue of autonomy. As babies grow they like to participate in feeding and become messy. Mothers who insist on feeding to prevent the messiness, deprive the child of learning and cause frustration and feeding difficulties. Problems may also arise due to inappropriate weaning practices.

C. *18 months — 3 years*: Weight gain decelerates in this age group. At the same time, linear growth accelerates. This results in decreasing appetite and the child appears to be thin instead of being chubby which causes anxiety to the parent. Urging the child to eat produces resistance and further anxiety to the parent. In severe feeding problems, the mother may have unconscious conflicts about nurturing.

Pica may be a presenting problem which may be due to mental retardation, neglect or nutritional deficiency.

D. *4–10 years*: The commonest complaint in this age group is that the child does not eat regular meals but has multiple snacks (biscuits, fast foods, cordials and soft drinks) in between meals.

E. *Adolescents*: Concern about weight is very common and the vast majority do not present to the medical profession. Those who are brought by their parents to the doctor may be "normal" or may be suffering from a variety of physical or psychological disorders. These children may conflict with their parents about eating but may not have problems or concerns about weight or body image. Where lack of eating is associated with weight loss, this may be due to psychiatric disorders (anorexia nervosa, depression, schizophrenia, conversion disorders), gastrointestinal disorders (e.g. Crohn's disease), endocrine disorders (e.g. diabetes mellitus) and malignancy (e.g. brain tumour). History in these cases has to be amplified after the physical examination.

Bulimia: Presents with binge eating usually followed by either self induced vomiting and/or the use of diuretics or laxatives, dieting or fasting or vigorous exercise in order to prevent weight gain. There may be a history of anorexia nervosa or weight may always have been within normal range though a pre-occupation with dieting and weight loss often precedes the disorder. A history of remissions and relapses is common.

Obesity: Many obese children are obese as infants and also have obese parents. Those who present to the physician are more likely to have psychological problems (depression and dysphoria) than obese subjects in the population. The psychological disturbances may be the cause or the result of the obesity.

Obesity results mainly from a net increase in calorie intake. Therefore dietary intake and level of activity has to be established accurately. Obesity due to endocrine causes is uncommon and the diagnosis is usually possible by physical examination.

EXAMINATION

The most important part of the physical examination is the plotting of physical parameters (both present and previous measurements) on centile charts. Children following their previous centile growth and whose height and weight fall on the same centile, do not have significant medical problems.

Infants below the age of 6 months should be examined carefully for physical (e.g. cleft palate) and neurological (cerebral palsy) abnormalities which may be the cause of their feeding difficulties. Evidence for nutritional deficiencies should be sought in all cases.

The mother's breasts should be examined for conditions which may result in difficulty (e.g. inverted nipples) in breastfeeding.

MANAGEMENT

The management of young infants with feeding problems can be very difficult because the parents often want a "quick fix". Physical and neurological problems, if present, should be treated appropriately. As in the majority of cases there is no physical abnormality, intervention is infant focused, parent focused or a mixture of both. In the former group, various behavioural therapies aim to extinguish maladaptive infant behaviours associated with feeding and to promote new adaptive feeding skills. Mother or father focused strategies aim at treating depression and anxiety, and supporting adaptive coping strategies, especially for those with personality difficulties. Interventions that target the parent–infant relationship, focus on perceived developmental and relationship problems, which are often rooted in the mother's past attachment problems. Thus some of these programmes will require introspection, while others deal with those who are resistant to such approaches, or who are less able to handle abstract problems.

An explanation of normal growth of infants and children and demonstration on centile charts that the child is growing normally will allay the anxiety of parents who are concerned that their child eats "nothing".

Children and adolescents with weight loss and obesity should be referred to a paediatrician for further assessment and treatment.

21 Enuresis

Enuresis literally means involuntary urination. Clinically, enuresis refers to children who have involuntary discharge of urine beyond the age they should have established bladder control. Children are not labelled enuretic unless the symptom persists beyond the age of 5 years.

HISTORY

The age of presentation will depend on the expectation of the parents. The higher social economic group of parents seek help at an earlier age and sometimes have unrealistic expectations. It is important to determine whether the enuresis is during the day or only at night, whether the child has never been dry or is this a new problem, what treatment has been offered and what are the results of the treatment and how well the child is motivated to succeed in remaining dry. In the case of a child who has achieved bladder control and has developed enuresis as a new problem, the physician should elicit problems that may have precipitated the enuresis. These include family break-up, separation, arrival of a new child as well as pathological conditions which increase frequency of micturation (urinary tract infection, diabetes mellitus). In the case of children who have never been dry, a developmental history is important. The vast majority of children are nocturnal enuretics and may have a family history of a similar disorder.

EXAMINATION

Physical examination usually shows no abnormality other than excoriation around the perineum in some patients. Examination of the abdomen should be carried out for renal masses, distended bladder and distended rectum. Blood pressure should be measured in all cases.

In patients with diurnal enuresis, a detailed neuro-developmental assessment should be carried out.

MANAGEMENT

In all patients with enuresis, a urinalysis should be carried out though in the majority of nocturnal enuretics, it will be normal. Urological investigations may be necessary in patients with daytime enuresis. Detailed neurological and urological investigations are indicated in diurnal enuresis.

Children under 5 years do not require any intervention other than reassurance of the child and the parents. In children above the age of 5 years a most important issue is the involvement of the child and his/her motivation in staying dry. In all cases the child should be encouraged, rewarded (not *bribed*) which could be in the form of stars, praise or occasionally, a present. Punitive measures such as scolding should be discouraged.

The best results are obtained by conditioning the child to respond to certain cues, such as a pad and bell. However, the child should be completely involved in the process otherwise it will result in failure. In this respect, motivation is all important. The child should be responsible for turning off the bell and turning it on when he/she goes to sleep.

Practical measures include using plastic pants or plastic draw sheets in order to help the mother cut down on her washing. It is important to emphasise to the child that this is not punishment but only facilitating the mother's work. Making the child feel guilty or ashamed will only exacerbate the problem.

Drugs that have been used in the management of nocturnal enuresis include imipramine and anti-diuretic hormones. They have limited value in the management and often result in relapses when the treatment is withdrawn.

Fluid restriction is of little value. Diurnal (night and day) enuresis will require bladder training.

22 Red Eye

Red eye can be caused by conjunctivitis, keratitis (inflammation of the cornea), iritis and glaucoma.

HISTORY

Depending on the aetiology, conjunctivitis is characterised by itchiness, mild discomfort, swelling of the eyelids and mucopurulent or serous discharge. In keratitis, the principal symptoms are a foreign body sensation in the eye, blepharospasm, photophobia, blurred vision and significant tearing. Iritis presents with photophobia and excessive tearing. Glaucoma presents with excessive tearing, blepharospasm, photophobia and pain (which may be manifested as irritability in infants) and progressive enlargement of the eye.

In addition to the eye symptoms, the child may present with symptoms of systemic disease (e.g. joint pain in rheumatoid arthritis) which may be the cause of the eye problems.

EXAMINATION

Patients with conjunctivitis have mucopurulent discharge. The eyelids are swollen and hyperemic. Corneal involvement can occur in conjunctivitis due to Herpes simplex, chlamydia, gonococcus and adenoviral infections leading to serious vision disturbances.

In keratitis there is perilimbal conjunctival injection (ciliary flush) which may be confused with conjunctivitis. The cornea may have hazy patches. Dendritic keratitis due to Herpes simplex virus infection can be demonstrated as a branching pattern by fluorescein staining.

As in keratitis, in iritis there is perilimbal conjunctival injection. Other eye signs include constricted or irregular pupil, "flare" in the aqueous humor, evidence of inflammatory deposits on the posterior surface of the cornea (keratic precipitates), congestion and sometimes neo-vascularisation of the iris. In chronic cases, there may be degenerative changes of the cornea and lenticular opacity (cataracts).

The major physical findings in glaucoma include increase in ocular pressure, corneal clouding and buphthalmos. Optic nerve atrophy and loss of vision may be found.

In all cases, a general physical examination should be carried out to exclude systemic diseases that have association with keratitis, iritis and glaucoma.

MANAGEMENT

The red eye due to conjunctivitis must be distinguished from that due to keratitis, iritis and glaucoma as the latter require urgent referral to an ophthalmologist. Allergy, bacteria and viruses can all cause conjunctivitis. Diagnosis can be made on clinical grounds. Microscopy and culture should be carried out in all newborn infants and those with severe conjunctivitis. Most patients with bacterial conjunctivitis are treated with topical chloromycetin eye drops. Failure to respond suggests a possible viral infection (adenovirus, chlamydia) or allergy. A recurrence after discontinuing treatment supports a diagnosis of naso-lachrymal duct obstruction.

24 Fever of Unknown Origin

There is no clear consensus on the exact definition of fever or pyrexia of unknown origin (FUO or PUO). It may be defined as an intermittent temperature of more than 38°C which has been present for two weeks or more and the history, physical examination and simple laboratory tests such as chest X-ray, blood count, blood culture and micro-urine fail to reveal the diagnosis. The main causes can be grouped into (a) microbial inflammatory diseases, (b) non-microbial inflammatory diseases (collagen disease or vasculitis), (c) malignant disease, and (d) miscellaneous conditions such as anhidrosis and dysautonomia.

HISTORY

The nature of the *fever*, its frequency and periodicity, duration and the levels of temperature should be noted. The fever should be documented by regular measurement of temperature. Fairly regular daily or twice daily spikes are more often associated with non-microbial inflammatory or malignant disease. Rigors with spiking fever suggest septicaemia or the presence of pus in the body. Non-specific symptoms include irritability, anorexia, weight loss, rashes, joint pains, abdominal pain and diarrhoea.

A history of recent exposure to illnesses or animals or of recent travel may assist in unravelling the problem. The exposure may have occurred during travel to endemic areas, contact with farm animals or medical procedures such as injections, and administration of blood products. The type of infection will vary widely according to the geographic region. Infections likely to present as fever of unknown origin include glandular fever, tuberculosis, typhoid fever, malaria, brucellosis, and HIV infection.

The physician should inquire about underlying disorders such as rheumatic heart disease, hyposplenism, immunodeficiency disorders, bone marrow depression, sickle cell disease, familial dysautonomia, and anhydrotic disorders (icthyosis, ectodermal dysplasia) which predispose to febrile episodes.

PHYSICAL EXAMINATION

At the outset, the physician should decide whether the patient is ill or not. Ill patients are apathetic, have evidence of weight loss and require admission to hospital for further investigations. The physical signs may be subtle or non-specific. Lymphadenopathy with or without hyperaemia of the pharynx should alert the physician to the possibility of glandular fever, cytomegalovirus infection, toxoplasmosis, leukemias and lymphomas. Skin rashes suggest a viral or collagen disease. Point tenderness on bones suggests osteomyelitis whereas generalised muscle tenderness suggests mycoplasma or collagen diseases. Joints must be examined for swelling, range of movement and tenderness. Abdominal tenderness and anal tags are seen in Crohn's disease. Lack of tears or absent corneal reflex and a smooth tongue are found in familial dysautonomia. Small tonsils or oral thrush may be a manifestation of an underlying immunodeficiency problem.

MANAGEMENT

Hospitalisation of the patient is useful as it allows the documentation of the fever pattern; furthermore, the clinician is able to evaluate the patient repeatedly. In some cases, transitory physical signs such as the evanescent rash of juvenile rheumatoid arthritis may only be documented after a period of observation. If the child looks well and is not deteriorating, a period of observation may yield new physical signs which would help in the diagnosis.

Investigations which may be helpful in making a diagnosis may include full blood count, erythrocyte sedimentation rate, chest X-ray, blood culture, urinalysis, skin tests (tuberculosis, mycosis) and special serological tests for diseases such as hepatitis, infectious mononucleosis, toxoplasmosis, cytomegalovirus infection, brucellosis and typhoid. Multiple blood cultures may be necessary to diagnose endocarditis or osteomyelitis. Gallium and CT scanning are invaluable in diagnosing osteomyelitis, abscess and malignancy.

25 The Floppy Infant

HISTORY

The problem may present at any age. In the newborn infant, important aspects of the history include polyhydramnios and decreased foetal movements *in utero*, perinatal history of cerebral birth trauma and drugs given to the mother, family history of specific motor disorders such as myasthenia gravis or myotonic dystrophy. In the older infant, the age of onset and the progress of the hypotonia should be determined. Additional problems include difficulties in sucking and swallowing, failure to thrive and frequent respiratory infections.

In many cases, the patient may present with symptoms of a primary disease in which hypotonia may be a prominent feature. These include weakness, delayed milestones, mental deficiency, involuntary movements, lax joints and contractures. In the newborn, respiratory muscle weakness may be severe enough to require respiratory support.

PHYSICAL EXAMINATION

Hypotonia should be suspected in any infant who assumes unusual postures, has decreased resistance to passive movements and demonstrates relative immobility. The infant may have excessive range of joint mobility or joint contractures. A detailed neurological examination (including developmental assessment) should be carried out to assess the integrity of the central nervous system and to establish the anatomic level of the neurological lesion. Additional findings, such as enlarged liver or dysmorphic features may give further clues to the diagnosis.

DIAGNOSIS

The first step is to establish the absence or presence of significant muscle weakness. Significant muscle weakness is not present if an infant can move spontaneously or raise an extremity against gravity. In such cases, the floppiness is due to pathology in the central nervous system or a systemic disorder such as connective tissue disorders, endocrinopathies, metabolic disorders or malnutrition. In the former, the deep tendon reflexes are preserved and there are other signs of central nervous system involvement, e.g. developmental delay, seizures.

Hypotonia with weakness is caused by diseases affecting the lower motor neurone unit (anterior horn cell, peripheral nerve, neuro-muscular junction, muscle). In these patients, deep tendon reflexes are depressed or absent.

In diseases of the anterior horn cell (Werdnig Hoffman disease, arthrogryphosis multiplex congenita, Pompe disease), an additional physical finding is fasciculation of the muscles. Other clinical features may distinguish these from each other, e.g. Werdnig-Hoffman disease is progressive in contrast to arthrogryphosis multiplex congenita, while Pompe disease is accompanied with cardiac failure, cardiac enlargement and hepatomegaly.

In diseases affecting the peripheral nerves (Charcot-Marie-Tooth disease, Guillain-Barre syndrome) the motor weakness begins in the distal muscles. Sensory loss may also be present. There may be an increase in cerebrospinal fluid protein and reduction in nerve conduction.

Fatigue with repetitive motor activity is characteristic of diseases of the neuromuscular junction (myasthenia gravis, botulism). These patients present with ocular palsies, feeding difficulties and respiratory paralysis. Paralysis of the limbs and depression of deep tendon reflexes are late signs. The muscle biopsy is normal. The diagnosis may be confirmed by appropriate neurophysiological and pharmacological tests.

Unlike peripheral neuropathies, myopathies affect proximal muscles first. These diseases are age specific and have characteristic clinical presentations. There is an increase in muscle enzymes (creatine phosphokinase). The diagnosis is confirmed by muscle biopsy which shows a particular myopathic pattern.

A simple approach to the diagnosis of a floppy infant is shown in the accompanying table.

	FLOPPY INFANT	
NO SIGNIFICANT WEAKNESS	CNS DISORDERS	(1) CEREBRAL PALSY
		(2) NON-SPECIFIC MENTAL RETARDATION
Deep tendon reflexes: Normal or Increased	(Mental retardation ±)	(3) SPECIFIC SYNDROMES (Down, Prader Willi)
		(4) STORAGE DISEASES (lipidosis, mucopoly-saccharidosis)
	CONNECTIVE TISSUE DISORDERS	Ehlers-Danlos syndrome Marfan syndrome
	ENDOCRINE DISORDERS	Hypothyroidism Hypopituitarism Cushing's syndrome
	METABOLIC DISORDERS (Hypoglycaemia, acidosis, FTT)	Fats Amino Acids Infantile hypercalcaemia Renal tubular acidosis
SIGNIFICANT MUSCLE WEAKNESS Deep Tendon Reflexes: Diminished	ANTERIOR HORN CELL Fasciculation +	Werdnig-Hoffman Arthrogryphosis Multiplex Congenita, Pompe
	PERIPHERAL NEUROPATHY (Distal involvement) (Sensory loss) (CSF protein up) (Nerve conduction down)	Guillain-Barre syndrome Charcot-Marie-Tooth Disease

(Cont'd)

NEUROMUSCULAR JUNCTION
(Most used muscles affected)   Myasthenia gravis
                                    Botulism

MUSCULAR DYSTROPHY
(Proximal involvement)   Dystrophia myotonica
(Creatine phosphokinase)   Duchenne (comes on late)
(Muscle biopsy abnormal)   Congenital myopathy
                                    Central core disease

MYOPATHIES
(Muscle biopsy abnormal)   Nemaline myopathy
                                    Mitochondrial myopathies

MYTONIA   Dystrophia myotonica

26 Ambiguous Genitalia

Genital development is completed in the first trimester. Female genital development is passive but a normally functioning ovary requires a 46XX karyotype. Atrophy of the Wolffian ducts and internal female genital development from the Muellerian duct will occur independent of hormones or genetic influences. In contrast, male genital differentiation is initiated at 3 different levels: (1) the sry gene located at chromosome Yp leads to testes development from the undifferentiated gonadal anlage; (2) the secretion of testosterone and anti-Muellerian hormone (AMH) from the newly formed testes leads to involution of the Muellerian anlage

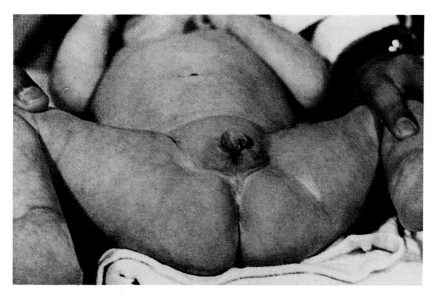

Fig. 26.1 Virilisation.

while testosterone supports male internal development from the Wolffian duct; (3) the external genitalia receives its male differentiation from dihydro-testosterone (DHT) which is produced by the cells of the external genitalia from testosterone. Adrenal or ectopic androgen production is not required for normal male development but excess will lead to virilisation of the female foetus (see Fig. 26.1).

HISTORY

Other than the abnormal anatomical abnormality, the newborn infant may have no other symptoms. In all cases, mothers should be asked about ingestion of drugs during pregnancy. Infants with ambiguous genitalia associated with congenital adrenal hyperplasia (Fig. 26.2) may develop severe vomiting with dehydration and/or failure to thrive in the first weeks of life. A family history of consanguity, infertility, unexplained neonatal deaths or anomalous genital differentiation should alert the physician to the diagnosis of congenital adrenal hyperplasia.

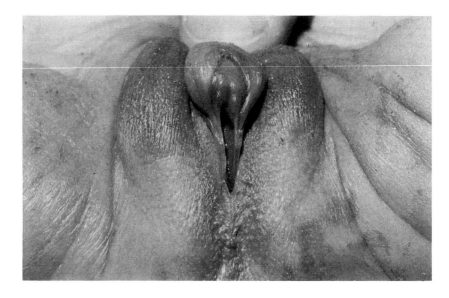

Fig. 26.2 Adrenogenital syndrome.

PHYSICAL EXAMINATION

General features which may help in the diagnosis of ambiguous genitalia include excess pigmentation (associated with ACTH), lymphoedema (associated with gonadal dysgeneses) and raised blood pressure (seen in 11-hydroxylase defect). Special attention should be given to the examination of the genitalia, their gross appearance and detailed anomalies. The physician should identify both the urethral and vaginal orifices. In many cases, the vagina has a common opening with the urethra (urogenital sinus). The urethral opening may be at the base of the clitoris which is so enlarged that it can be mistaken for a penis with a hypospadias. There may be no gonads palpable in the "scrotum" which may suggest a diagnosis of "undescended testis" in an infant who is female, as sometimes the urogenital sinus may extend to the tip of the phallus and the genitalia resemble those of a cryptorchid male.

In all newborns, a rectal examination is mandatory because during the first 48 hours of life, the uterus is firm and can be easily palpated. An ambiguous genitalia with unilateral cryptorchidism suggests gonadal asymmetry.

In the unrecognised patient with congenital adrenal hyperplasia, masculinisation progresses in the female infant and manifests by the development of pubic and axillary hair prematurely and acne. The voice assumes a masculine quality. These girls are muscular, and have a body build of a boy.

MANAGEMENT

In the neonate, assignment of the correct sex to the infant is a social emergency. The assignment of sex rearing, which is based largely on the possibilities for the correction of the ambiguous genitalia (and not on the chromosomal constitution) should be settled as early in life as possible. The presence of a uterus suggests that the infant will fare better with a female gender assignment regardless of other findings. The additional knowledge of the karyotype will facilitate the planning of further investigations and help in the differential diagnosis (Fig. 26.3).

Newborn 46XX with uterus. If laboratory studies (elevated 17-hydroxyprogesterone) suggest congenital adrenal hyperplasia, treat

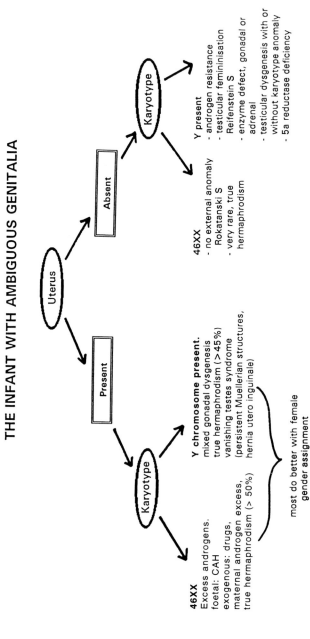

THE INFANT WITH AMBIGUOUS GENITALIA

Uterus

Present

Absent

Karyotype

Karyotype

46XX
Excess androgens.
foetal: CAH
exogenous: drugs,
maternal androgen excess,
true hermaphrodism (> 50%)

Y chromosome present.
mixed gonadal dysgenesis
true hermaphrodism (>45%)
vanishing testes syndrome
(persistent Muellerian structures,
hernia utero inguinale)

most do better with female
gender assignment

46XX
- no external anomaly
  Rokatanski S
- very rare, true
  hermaphrodism

Y present
- androgen resistance
- testicular femininisation
  Reifenstein S
- enzyme defect, gonadal or
  adrenal
- testicular dysgenesis with or
  without karyotype anomaly
- 5α reductase deficiency

Fig. 26.3

with cortisol and florinef replacement. In other cases, correct vaginal opening and recess phallus within the first year of life. Surgery has to be individualised according to findings and basic defect.

Newborn with uterus and some Y material on karyotype. The dysgenetic testes may look normal and produce normal gonadotropins and HCG response during early infancy. These testes are pre-malignant, not functional by adolescence and growth potential in patients with XY/XO mosaicism is very poor. The gonads should be removed and the patient is reared as a female.

Males with persistent Muellerian ducts often have autosomal recessive gene defect. Early excision of Muellerian structure may be difficult without damaging the spermatic duct.

46XX without detectable uterus is an exceedingly rare form of true hermaphrodism. Presence of vagina will provide a clue to the diagnosis. Other similar constellation are not associated with ambiguous external genital development.

Y chromosome and no uterus frequently presents with no ambiguous external genitalia but bilateral, gonad containing hernias. The hernias should be repaired and the gonads removed but only after hormonal stimulation and androgen receptor studies have provided insight into the genetic defect. The physical examination does not allow differentiation between androgen receptor defect, 51α reductase deficiency (cannot convert testosterone to dihydro-testosterone), and 17OH ketoreductase, or 20/21 hydroxylase deficiency. Complete forms should receive female gender assignment. Patients with gonadal dysgenesis due to mosaic karyotype (i.e. 46XY, 47XYY, 46X) will respond to testosterone therapy but may end up short in stature.

27 Goitre

HISTORY

Goitre may be present at birth. The mother should be asked about ingestion of anti-thyroid drugs, medications containing iodine and a history of hyperthyroidism (Graves disease). Most of these patients have no other symptoms though in some cases the enlarged thyroid may occasionally cause respiratory distress.

In older children, the enlarged thyroid is often symptomless. Some patients complain of mild discomfort upon palpation or swallowing.

It is essential to ascertain whether the symptoms of hyper- or hypothyroidism are present. Hyperthyroidism is suggested by irritability, erratic emotional outbursts, high food intake, nocturia, heat intolerance, accelerated linear growth and poor school performance. Hypothyroidism is slow in onset and symptoms may not be obvious. Cessation of growth, low food intake, poor school performance and "good behaviours", cold intolerance and constipation may be present.

Some patients treated for prolonged periods with iodine preparations develop goitres. Simple or colloid goitre is seen in pubescent girls who have normal thyroid function. Family history often reveals other members who have thyroid or auto-immune disease, diabetes or chromosomal disorders.

PHYSICAL EXAMINATION

Height or length, weight and past records of these patients require charting and may indicate cessation or acceleration of growth unless the patients are euthyroid. Inspection of the thyroid gland during swallowing is informative. In health, the thyroid gland is not visible. The right lobe is slightly larger than the left, is smooth and has a regular even surface. A very small paratracheal lymph node (delphian node) suggests auto-immunity rather than malignancy; however, a firm, rapidly enlarging gland with unilateral or even bilateral lymphadenopathy is a typical finding in thyroid malignancy.

Chronic lymphocytic thyroiditis (Hashimoto's disease) (Fig. 27.1), the most frequent cause of goitre, is characterised by a rubbery thyroid with cobblestone surface. Single thyroid nodules without accompanying lymphadenopathy usually represent benign foetal adenomas which are often cystic. Rapid painful thyroid enlargement after trauma is characteristic of haemorrhage into such a cyst.

Simple goitre may be large or small. It is firm in consistency, may be asymmetric or nodular and may become mullinodular. It is something difficult to differentiate from chronic lymphocytic thyroiditis.

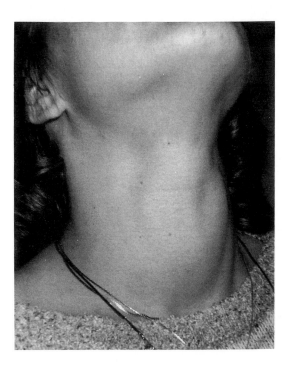

Fig. 27.1 Goitre due to Hashimoto's disease.

MANAGEMENT

The most important initial evaluation is to determine whether euthyroidism, hyper- or hypothyroidism is present (TSH and Free T_4). Simultaneously serum thyroid tissue antibodies suggesting an autoimmune disease process should be measured. Thyroid ultrasound might provide information suggestive but not diagnostic of the aetiology of the goitre. An isotope thyroid uptake and scan will distinguish between a hot, cold and "warm" thyroid nodule according to its participation in thyroid hormone synthesis.

Therapy is entirely dependent on the diagnosis and the endocrine status of the patient. In the presence of hypothyroidism, prompt treatment is essential. In cosmetically distractive goitres, surgical treatment may be indicated to reduce glandular size. Hyperthyroidism is treated either with radioactive iodine, antithyroid drugs or rarely with surgery. The approach to thyroid nodules depends on the results of the biopsy: benign nodules do not have to be removed surgically; hot nodules which have very high isotope uptake while simultaneously suppressing uptake in the rest of the gland, will respond very well to radioactive iodine therapy.

and phase of respiration. At the apex, the innocent systolic murmur (Still's murmur) is low pitched and has a musical ("seagull") quality. At the base, it is high pitched and blowing. In the neck, it is very short and early and can be heard over the supraclavicular region.

MANAGEMENT

It is important to be able to reassure the family when the heart is structurally normal, that the murmur is innocent, that restrictions or precautions are not necessary. The child should be discharged from follow-up. Children suspected to have a pathological murmur should be referred to a specialist cardiac unit for further evaluation.

30 Hyperactivity

HISTORY

Hyperactivity is not a unitary condition. Symptoms vary with different times and situations and also with age. The hyperactive child may run all the time in the preschool years, may not be able to sit quietly in a chair in early school grades and may be fidgety in adolescent and adult years. It may also be a symptom of a variety of other clinical disorders. Often hyperactivity is the presenting symptom of attention deficit hyperactivity disorder (ADHD).

When a child is referred for hyperactivity the interview with the parents clarifies the quality of hyperactivity, its age of onset and duration, the situations in which it occurs, coincidental characteristics, e.g. disruptiveness and what circumstances make it worse or better. A medical history includes inquiring about the child's vision and hearing. Inquiry is made about whether the child is in an appropriate learning situation. Family stresses and parental disorders will also be relevant, e.g. marital and parenting disagreements and parental depression. Disciplinary strategies and current handling of the hyperactivity or restlessness are explored. The parents' sense of efficacy and control (the possibility of abuse should be borne in mind) should be determined. The child may be able to give information about his perception of the problem and what might have caused it and convey his feelings and friendships and possible concurrent problems, e.g. depression. Family interviews may illuminate siblings' perceptions of family relationships.

Children with ADHD are typically referred to the physician in the preschool and school years. The hyperactivity has an off-task, disruptive quality. The child's poor attention span contributes to poor schoolwork and poor peer relationships (often because of wanting to do something else, disruptiveness and inability to wait turns at games). However attention may diverge sharply between boring and enjoyable activities. Distractibility is also often present and impulsivity is pervasive in social and learning situations. A developmental inquiry may elicit different findings at different ages: a history of extreme restlessness, colic and an aversion to being cuddled in early infancy; incessant activity requiring intense supervision, an unawareness of other children's feelings and often temper tantrums and aggression in preschool children; and increasing effects on many areas of the child's life (especially in the areas of cognitive and social development, self-esteem regulation and depression) in middle childhood and adolescence.

EXAMINATION

The child may not be restless at the first visit, often due to anxiety about attendance. Family interaction should be observed: for instance, parents may interact with the hyperactive child in an intrusive and controlling way. Reports should be sought from multiple sources (parents, child and teachers). The child's cognitive functioning and grade levels should be assessed. Specialised testing for learning disabilities may be needed.

DIAGNOSIS

There is still considerable variability in making the diagnosis of ADHD. The likelihood of making a positive diagnosis varies with the number of sources consulted. If parents, teachers, child and physician are all required to make the diagnosis, the prevalence is much lower than if only one source is required. However some physicians only make the diagnosis if the syndrome is pervasive (i.e. occurs in more than one situation, e.g. home and school).

Many children with ADHD may also have oppositional conduct and learning disorders; and hyperactive children when presented for the former diagnosis may in fact have the latter instead. Conduct and oppositional disorders may be associated with restlessness and inattention due to the lack of motivation at school. The ADHD symptoms are mild and secondary to the main conduct or oppositional problems. Learning difficulties may also present with restlessness and lack of attention at school, which is due to a mismatch between the child's capacities and the school situation. Children with adjustment problems, especially boys, may also be restless and inattentive in relation to identifiable psychosocial stressors. Lastly and commonly, some parents and teachers do not know what to expect in terms of activity for children at different ages, especially boys, and symptoms may be within normal limits.

MANAGEMENT

The details of intervention in hyperactivity will depend on the diagnosis, but intervention will need to be multi-focussed (educational, psychological, familial and possibly pharmacological).

Non-pharmacological treatments include behavioural therapy, cognitive and social skills training, remedial education, parent training, family therapy and individual child therapy; these may be combined in an individualised comprehensive treatment programme. Dietary alterations may be of use in a small number of cases; however, the evidence for such measures is anecdotal.

Stimulants have proved to be effective in treatment in numerous controlled trials. However they should be used with caution as many side effects have been recorded.

Hyperactivity associated with conduct and oppositional disorders, depression and learning difficulties (which are diagnosed on the basis of the symptom profiles) also requires multi-modal non-drug treatment. Conduct disordered children with hyperactivity or brain dysfunction may respond to stimulant medication, though those with different concomitant disorders such as epilepsy and psychosis will each require a different sort of pharmacological intervention. As with ADHD, medication will not suffice in itself.

In some cases, parents may be reassured that the hyperactivity is within normal limits. In this situation and also in the case of ADHD, it is useful to find an activity that channels the child's energy and for which he can potentially achieve acclaim and foster supporting relationships.

31 Immunisation Schedule

AGE	VACCINE	COMMENTS
Birth	BCG	In high endemic and high risk groups
	Hepatitis B	
2 Months	DPT, OPV, Hib Hepatitis B	
4 Months	DPT, OPV, Hib	
6 Months	DPT, OPV, Hib Hepatitis B	
12 Months	MMR	Earlier in high endemic areas
18 Months	DPT, OPV, Hib	May be given at 15 months with MMR if low compliance
5 Years	CDT, MMR	Preferably before entry to primary school
15 Year	ADT	Preferably before leaving secondary school

Repeat thereafter every 10 years

Abbreviations used:

ADT: Adult type diphtheria and tetanus toxoid,
BCG: Bacille Calmette-Guerin,
CDT: Combined diphtheria and tetanus toxoid,
DPT: Diphtheria, Pertussis and Tetanus toxoid,
Hib: *Haemophilus influenzae* type B vaccine,
MMR: Measles mumps and Rubella vaccine,
OPV: Sabin oral (trivalent) Polio Vaccine,

NOTES:

1. Interruption of the recommended schedule does not require restarting the entire immunisation schedule. Immunisation should proceed from the time it was interrupted.

2. Un-immunised children under the age of 5 years should receive full immunisations except that the schedule is modified. The schedule and number of Hib vaccine (0–3) depend on age at first dose and which Hib vaccine is used.

2(a) In Australia, pertussis vaccine is not "approved for use beyond 3 years and 11 months".

3. For BCG vaccination other than in neonates, Mantoux test is mandatory.

4. Children over the age of 5 years do not require immunisation against *Haemophilus influenzae* type B.

5. Mild illnesses (upper respiratory tract infection, diarrhoea) are not contraindications for immunisation. Immunisation should be deferred for children with high fever until their illness is resolved.

COMPLICATIONS AND CONTRAINDICATIONS

Diphtheria and Tetanus: mild fever, local pain, redness and swelling.

Pertussis: Local tenderness, fever, irritability, lethargy, convulsions, hypotonia, hyporesponsiveness (1:2000), encephalopathy (1:100 000) permanent neurologic sequelae (rare). Contraindications are previous *severe* reaction to pertussis vaccine, unstable or progressive neurological disorder, microbiologically confirmed infection. Family history of neurological disease or a static neurological lesion is not a contraindication for pertussis immunisation.

Measles: Fever and rash are the common complications. Contraindications are pregnancy, high fever, anaphylactic (not just "allergy") reaction to eggs, immunodeficiency.

Mumps: Fever, rash, seizures and encephalitis (instance is less than expected in general population). Contraindications as with measles.

Rubella: Rash, lymphadenopathy, arthralgia. Contraindications as with measles.

Hepatitis B: Local tenderness, neurological adverse reaction rarely occurs.

BCG: Localised lymphadenopathy, disseminated tuberculosis (rare).

32 The Child with Recurrent Infection

HISTORY

Most children with recurrent infections present in the context of respiratory tract symptoms which include rhinorrhoea, nasal obstruction, cough, wheeze with or without low grade fever which are very frequently due to allergy. Eliciting of other atopic symptoms such as eczema, or urticaria, or a family history of eczema, hay fever and asthma can be helpful. Some of these children have recurrent otitis media and may have had insertion of ventilation tubes for secretory otitis media (glue ear). Other conditions which predispose to recurrent respiratory tract infections include parental smoking, attendance at day care nursery, small children with older siblings, inadequate treatment of a bacterial infection or underlying disease process (Table 32.1). In the latter case, the child may also have symptoms of the primary disease — failure to thrive or chronic diarrhoea in cystic fibrosis, history of episode of coughing and choking in toddler with foreign body aspiration, infections at other sites in immunodeficiency states. The family history may be very helpful since many immunodeficiencies in childhood are X-linked.

PHYSICAL EXAMINATION

In the assessment of the patient with recurrent infections, the weight and height measurements are very useful in assessing the severity and the chronicity of the infection. The infections can be more readily recognised by clear objective findings (thrush, herpetic lesions, purulent

**Table 32.1 The Child with Recurrent Infection:
Disease processes associated with infection**

DISEASE PROCESS	EXAMPLE
Systemic disease	Diabetes mellitus
Foreign body	Bronchial, nasal, prosthesis
Obstructive	Urinary tract
Portal of entry	Skin disease, CSF leak
Respiratory disease	Cystic fibrosis, asthma, Eustachian tube dysfunction
Congenital heart disease	L to R shunt
Secondary immunodeficiency	Malnutrition, prematurity
Primary immunodeficiency	X-linked hypogammaglobulinaemia

discharge, chest signs, meningitis, abscesses). Signs of atopy include clear nasal discharge, hypertrophic nasal mucosa, rhonchi in chest and evidence of skin atopy. The examination may elicit findings (Table 32.2) which together with the history will assist in the diagnosis of specific immunodeficiency disorders.

MANAGEMENT

When a child presents with the complaint of frequent infections, the initial questions to be addressed include:

1. Are the symptoms likely to be due to infection?
2. Are the episodes unusual in their number, severity or frequency?

Table 32.2 Primary Immunodeficiency (ID): Clues to diagnosis

CLINICAL FEATURE	ID IN WHICH PRESENT
Facial abnormalties	di George syndrome
Heart disease, neonatal tetany	di George syndrome
Ataxia, conjunctival telangiectasia	Ataxia telangiectasia
Eczema, petechiae	Wiskott-Aldrich syndrome
Mouth ulcers, neutropenia	ID with hyper-IgM
Absent tonsils	X-linked hypogammaglobulinaemia
Nail dystrophy	Mucocutaneous candidiasis
Thrush, failure-to-thrive	Severe combined immunodeficiency
Purulent sinopulmonary infection	Hypogammaglobulinaemia

3. Is there likely to be an underlying disorder contributing to the occurrence?

In assessing the frequency and severity of infection, one has to take into account the age of the child and the parent's response to their child's illness. Infections occur quite frequently in young healthy children (Table 32.3). Parents vary in the likelihood that they will seek advice about normal childhood infections, e.g. a mother in full-time employment may be more concerned about the impact on the family when infections disrupt schooling or care arrangements.

A sweat test is necessary for a diagnosis of cystic fibrosis.

Table 32.3 Expected Frequency of Infections in Childhood

AGE (YEARS)	INFECTIONS/YEAR
<1	6
1–2	6
3–4	5
5–9	4
10–14	3

**Table 32.4 Primary Immunodeficiency in Children:
Screening tests**

Blood count

Immunoglobulins G, A, M

Antibody responses to previous vaccines
Tetanus, measles, polio

Isoagglutinins (anti-A, anti-B)

For diagnosis of immunodeficiency, a few simple investigations may provide a diagnosis or indicate further appropriate studies (Table 32.4). Lymphopaenia is often present in severe combined immunodeficiency and other cellular defects, and hypogammaglobulinaemia is prevalent in the former (though IgG level may be normal in early infancy). Lymphocyte phenotyping will identify most T cell disorders. Other investigations may be necessary in order to make a correct diagnosis. Antibody production disorders respond well to IgG replacement. Severe combined immunodeficiency can almost always be corrected by bone marrow transplantation. A compatible sibling donor is not essential, but the key to success is early diagnosis.

33 Inguino-Scrotal Swellings in Childhood

The main inguino-scrotal swellings in childhood include hernias, hydrocoeles, undescended testes, torsion of the testis and its appendages, varicocoeles and tumours.

HISTORY

The swellings may be observed by parents or found on routine examination. Hydrocoeles can vary in size but do so very slowly and do not disappear when palpated. Pain is the prominent symptom in torsion of the testis. Though there may be some discomfort, pain is not a feature of a hydrocoele, uncomplicated hernia or a tumour. In strangulated hernia, there may also be symptoms of acute intestinal obstruction.

EXAMINATION

Both hernias and hydrocoeles have the same pathophysiology, i.e. a patent processus vaginalis. In hydrocoeles, the communication is so small that only fluid passes from the peritoneal cavity to the scrotum, whereas with hernias, communication is large enough to permit bowel to pass into the inguinal canal and the sac. Both hernias and hydrocoeles transilluminate well in infants and as such, this sign is of limited value.

Hydrocoeles are soft or tense, fluctuate in size and can become quite large with an intercurrent illness. As the fluid is contained within the processus vaginalis, it is possible to get above the swelling. Inguinal hernias in infancy are usually indirect and therefore must come through the inguinal canal rings. It is impossible, therefore, to get above the swelling. It may be possible to reduce the hernia and sometimes feel gurgling in the swelling.

If no inguino-scrotal swelling is present at the time of the examination but there is a good history of one being present, then this swelling will almost certainly be a hernia. A thickened cord on one side may be the only objective sign of the presence of an inguinal hernia that has reduced.

A scrotal swelling in an older child may be due to a varicocoele. These feel like a "bag of worms" in the scrotum. The patient should be examined standing up to look for this sign, as the distended veins collapse when lying down.

The scrotum is red, often tender and quite oedematous in patients with torsion of the testis. Testicular tumours can be recognised by their hard consistency without tenderness.

Inguinal swellings may be due to a hydrocoele of the cord which is a loculated and localised collection of fluid along the cord within the processus vaginalis. It feels like an extra testicle (firm and mobile). In little girls, an inguinal swelling which is mobile, firm and elliptical in shape is due to a hernia of the ovary which is rarely damaged but may become quite oedematous.

Lymph nodes in the groin are very common and sometimes cause confusion, but unlike inguinal hernias, they lie inferior to the inguinal ligament. However, they may be difficult to distinguish from femoral hernias which are very rare in children. Undescended testicles can be confused with hernias but unlike hernias, they do not fluctuate in size, so a fluctuating inguinal swelling with an undescended testis is a hernia.

MANAGEMENT

Inguinal hernias require early operation and the younger the child, the more likely it is to become strangulated. A strangulated hernia requires an urgent operation.

Hydrocoeles do not require treatment in infants, as 95% will resolve spontaneously by the age of 2–3 years. If persistent, they require operation for cosmetic reasons and the possible risk of developing a hernia.

Varicocoeles do not usually require operation unless they cause symptoms.

Tests are usually not required in the diagnosis of inguino-scrotal swellings other than when a tumour is suspected. In such cases, tumour markers, CT scans and nuclear imaging are usually required.

34 Jaundice

Clinically, jaundice is manifested by a yellow discolouration of skin and mucous membranes. Age and associated symptoms are important factors in assessment and management.

HISTORY

Neonatal Jaundice — may present within the first 24 hours of life, or may appear at the age of 2–3 days or may persist beyond the first week of life.

1. *Jaundice appearing within the first 24 hours of birth* is often due to haemolysis or congenital infections.

   1.1. *History*: The physician should obtain information on the mother's blood group, antibodies during pregnancy, previously affected babies, infections during pregnancy, family history of haemolysis, anaemia, gestation and birth weight, duration of labour and ruptured membranes, time of cord clamping.

   1.2. *Physical Examination*: Look for colour, external bruising, rashes (petechiae, blueberry muffins), head circumference, cataracts, choroidoretinitis, hepatosplenomegaly and dysmorphic features.

   1.3. *Management*: All infants require serum bilirubin measurement (total and direct), full blood count, peripheral blood film, blood group and Coomb's test. The patient suspected of having congenital infections will require serological tests (TORCH screen). Appropriate cultures (blood, urine, CSF) need to be carried out in suspected acquired infections. Treatment will depend on aetiology, presence of anaemia or other problems (cardiac failure, respiratory distress) and level of bilirubin (phototherapy or exchange transfusion).

2. *Onset of jaundice at the age of 3 Days*

2.1. Majority of cases are physiological, have no physical symptoms and signs other than jaundice.

2.2. *Management*: Most infants require no investigations other than measurement of serum bilirubin. Further investigations are required if the rate of rise is greater than 100 mmol/l/24 hours; total bilirubin is more than 250 mmol/l in full term infants; and more than 200 mmol/l in pre-term infants; the jaundice shows no evidence of abating by the age of 7 days; and direct (conjugated) bilirubin is more than 10% of total bilirubin. Jaundice that recurs is always pathological. The possible explanations for physiological jaundice are increased bilirubin load or decreased elimination of bilirubin from plasma.

Hyperbilirubinaemia may require intervention as it has been associated with bilirubin toxicity (high tone deafness, learning difficulties, kernicterus). There is no bilirubin level that can be used for intervention in all infants which depends on gestation period, birth weight and age of the infant. Other factors that have to be taken into consideration are hypoxia, acidosis, hypothermia and infection, all of which predispose to bilirubin toxicity. Furthermore, the rate of rise of bilirubin is important in planning when to intervene. Treatment modalities that are available include phototherapy, exchange transfusion and phenobarbitone. Phenobarbitone works very slowly and its effect is not apparent for nearly 48 hours. It is not much use for rapid lowering of the serum bilirubin but it may be useful in communities where there is a high incidence of hyper-bilirubinaemia when it can be given to mothers prior to delivery. Exchange transfusion is indicated when it is necessary to urgently lower the serum bilirubin. In most other cases phototherapy would be the treatment of choice.

Recognised side effects of phototherapy include loose stools, rashes, increased fluid loss, and hypothermia. Bronzing of the skin (Bronze baby syndrome) has been described in cases where phototherapy has been used in infants having high conjugated (direct reacting) bilirubin.

3. *Jaundice in an infant more than 2 weeks old*

3.1. *History*: Pregnancy with particular reference to infections and drug intake. Family history of jaundice, gestation period, birth weight, type of feeding, any feeding problems, change of weight since birth, time of onset of jaundice (increasing or decreasing), colour of urine and stools.

3.2. *Physical examination*: Colour, jaundice (severity, yellow or tinge of green). Evidence of congenital infection: Cataracts, hepatosplenomegaly, rashes, head circumference, heart murmurs.

Brief neurological examination: Suck, grasp and Moro reflexes.

3.3. *Management*: The most important investigation is the serum bilirubin level (total and direct).

3.3.1. If serum bilirubin is mainly indirect (e.g. total serum bilirubin 300 μmol/l with a direct of 20 μmol/l), likely diagnoses are breast milk jaundice, hypothyroidism and mild haemolytic anaemias. Obtain result of neonatal thyroid screening test. Breast milk jaundice requires no treatment other than reassurance to mother. If mother is worried, then the diagnosis needs to be confirmed. Suspension (*not stopping*) of breastfeeding for 48 hours will lower the serum bilirubin rapidly. Breastfeeding may be continued after demonstration that the jaundice is breast milk jaundice.

3.3.2. Conjugated hyperbilirubinaemia (i.e. raised direct serum bilirubin, e.g. total bilirubin 150 μmol/l, direct bilirubin 100 μmol/l) may be due to a variety of very important and sometimes life-threatening disorders such as infections, galactosaemia and biliary atresia which require immediate assessment and treatment.

4. *Jaundice in older children*

4.1. ***History***: In this age group, unconjugated hyperbilirubinaemia (acholuric jaundice — urine contains no bile) is an uncommon presenting symptom and is usually due to haemolytic anaemias. The patient may present with pallor or other manifestations of the disease causing the haemolysis. Gilbert's syndrome is the main hepatic cause of unconjugated hyperbilirubinaemia. These patients have exacerbation of the jaundice during times of stress, particularly infections.

Conjugated hyperbilirubinaemia (pale stools, urine contains bile) is mainly due to one form or another of hepatitis. Very occasionally gall stones, choledochal cysts, cholangitis and inflammatory bowel disease may be associated with jaundice. The presenting symptoms may include nausea, poor appetite, abdominal pain, abdominal lump and fever. Pruritus may be a prominent feature.

4.2. ***Examination***: Besides jaundice, the patient will manifest physical findings of the primary disease, e.g. splenomegaly in haemolytic anaemias, liver enlargement and tenderness in hepatitis A, lymph node enlargement in infectious mononucleosis, and a lump in choledochal cysts. The presence of ascites indicates a more serious hepatic insufficiency.

4.3. ***Management***: Liver function tests will usually clarify if there is underlying liver disease or not. Relatively normal hepatocellular enzymes (ALT/SGPT, AST/SGOT) associated with elevation of gamma GT and the liver component of alkaline phosphatase, would suggest that the problem is primarily obstructive. On the other hand, high levels of the former enzymes would suggest hepatitis. Ultrasound of the liver and biliary tree has largely replaced oral or intravenous cholecystograms in the diagnosis of biliary problems. Needle liver biopsy may be necessary in selected cases. In haemolytic jaundice, other than the raised indirect bilirubin, the liver function tests would be normal.

The haemolytic anaemias may require blood transfusions and corticosteroids. Patients with hepatocellular disease require supportive therapy. Patients with obstructive jaundice (conjugated hyperbilirubinaemia) may require specific surgical treatment to alleviate the obstruction. Phenobarbitone will lower unconjugated hyperbilirubin levels by facilitating excretion by stimulating bile water flow with its choleretic effect. Cholestyramine can also be effective by increasing bile flow and may be useful in some cases. Extra fat soluble vitamins are necessary because of the relative lack of bile. In infancy, it may also be necessary to use special infant formulas in which the long chain fat has been replaced with medium chain triglycerides (MCT) as the latter do not need bile for absorption.

35 Joint Pain

Joint pain may be due to arthralgia or arthritis. The latter term implies inflammation, whereas the former refers to a sensation of pain.

HISTORY

Joint pain in a young child can be inferred from the patient's refusal to move a given extremity or joint. It can be sudden in onset or be insidious over days or weeks. Sudden onset with a history of a fall or direct blow to the joint suggests a traumatic aetiology. In patients with a coagulation disorder, e.g. haemophilia, history of trauma may be difficult to elicit as minor trauma (which the patient may have forgotten) can precipitate the bleeding into the joint. The presence of fever points towards an infective process such as septic arthritis or acute viral infection, a rheumatic disease such as juvenile rheumatoid arthritis or a systemic disease. Other symptoms which may help in the diagnosis include the number of joints involved, the type of joints involved, rash, mucous membrane involvement, lymph node enlargement and the presence of symptoms of chronic diseases (such as inflammatory bowel disease) which can involve the joints.

EXAMINATION

In arthralgia the joints show no deformity though movement may be limited because of pain. In arthritis, the clinical features will depend on whether the condition is acute or chronic. In acute cases the joint shows redness, warmth, swelling which may be minimal (filling up of the contours of the joint) or severe. In chronic cases there is thickening of the synovial membrane, limitation of joint movements due to contractures and muscle atrophy. The latter may be seen within a few weeks of onset of the illness. In addition the skin may show dystrophic changes.

Both active and passive movements of the joint are limited which is in contrast to pain due to diseases of the bone adjacent to a joint. Examination of eyes in chronic cases may show iritis or keratitis.

DIAGNOSIS AND MANAGEMENT

Other than acute rheumatic fever, in rheumatic diseases of childhood there is some degree of joint deformity. Large joint involvement occurs in juvenile rheumatoid arthritis, ankylosing spondylitis, Reiter syndrome, psoriasis, systemic lupus erythematosus, dermatomyositis, polymyositis, scleroderma and mixed connective tissue disease. Small joint involvement is classically seen in rheumatoid arthritis (Figs. 35.1 and 35.2) which can also present as fever of unknown origin,

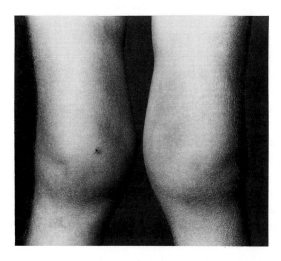

Fig. 35.1 *Rheumatoid arthritis* showing deformity of knees.

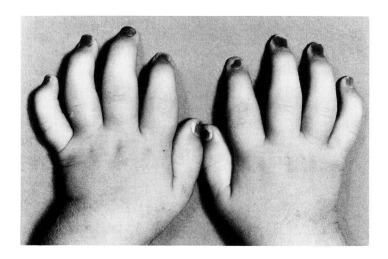

Fig. 35.2 *Polyarticular rheumatoid arthritis* involving the fingers of both hands.

lymphadenopathy and an evanescent rash. Each of these conditions has its own distinguishing features as seen on the clinical signs and symptoms and in the laboratory findings. They all tend to be chronic.

Joint pain caused by infections is acute in onset and short in duration if treated appropriately. Infections may be bacterial (*S. aureus, H. influenzae, N. gonorrhoeae* and *N. meningitidis*) or viral (rubella, mumps, chicken pox, adenovirus, Epstein-Barr virus, hepatitis A virus). The presence of systemic signs and symptoms of a viral infection or a recent history of MMR immunisation will help to make a diagnosis.

Inflammatory bowel disease can present with pain alone or inflammation as well of the large joints. The activity of the bowel disease may or may not correlate with exacerbation of joint symptoms. Connective tissue disorders, e.g. Marfan syndrome can present with joint pains as can many haematological disorders such as Henoch-Schonlein purpura, haemophilia, leukaemia and sickle cell disease. Hyperuricaemia due to leukaemia, haemolytic anaemia and Lesch-Nyhan syndrome can also present with joint pain.

Physical abuse must be considered in any joint injury if the history is incompatible with the physical findings.

The aim of treatment in the rheumatoid diseases is to relieve pain and maintain the normal range of joint movement. Medications include non-steroidal inflammatory drugs including salicylates, gold, hydroxychloroquine, D-penicillamine and methotrexate. Steroids may be necessary in resistant cases. The patient's eyes should be examined by an ophthalmologist for evidence of iritis and keratitis. Surgery is employed for joint reconstruction and release of contractures. In addition, all issues of chronic diseases in children need to be addressed.

36 Learning Problems

HISTORY

The child is most commonly referred by the parents or the teacher but sometimes by the family physician. The ensuing assessment will generally be multidisciplinary and may include all or some of the following: teacher, school and special education counsellors, general practitioner, paediatrician, neurologist, speech and occupational therapists, psychologist, psychiatrist, as well as child and family.

There is no typical clinical picture: the child may be referred because of aggression, problems with "on-task" behaviour in class, anxiety or depressive symptoms, a variety of physical complaints, or the learning problem may be the primary problem presented. In the last case, possible presenting complaints are very varied and may include: failure to complete work, specific weaknesses in academic skills, specific oral or written language problems, poor learning strategies, memory problems, untidiness and disorganisation, neuropsychological problems, physical performance problems including poor handwriting, poor motivation, work not in keeping with abilities and difficulties with the curriculum or teaching. If a learning problem is suspected, questions about the child's academic capacities and suitability for his current class environment are to be forefront.

The clinical history elicits information about school performance and ability in each academic area. Particular attention is paid to the child's developmental history, the child's attitude to school and the parents' attitude to the child, work and school. The child's handedness should be ascertained. There also may be a family history of learning disabilities. The time course of the disorder should be traced in order to unravel the relationships between the learning problem and the emotional, social and family difficulties which often present. The learning problem may have been present since the beginning of school, often pointing to intellectual or chronic socio-emotional factors, or of more recent onset often indicating a reaction to negative life events. Regardless of whether the accompanying difficulties are primary or secondary, they often require treatment in their own right.

The medical history should consider the following possible contributors: developmental immaturity for age (e.g. with low or very low birth weight children; children who are young for their peer group); sensory deficits and handicaps; diseases of the central nervous system (e.g. cerebral palsy, spina bifida, infections of the central nervous system, trauma, post-irradiation); chronic illness and other major handicaps; and nutritional deficits and sleep disorders (e.g. sleep apnoea).

The psychiatric and social history should consider: the child whose temperament (whether "difficult to handle" or "slow to warm up") does not fit the class situation; attention deficit disorder, which is frequently associated with academic underachievement; anxiety, depression or psychosis (the last of these rarely presenting as a learning problem); adolescent "acting out" against school (often learning difficulties have preceded this); delinquency in adolescence; insufficient social opportunity to learn ("lack of stimulation"); excessive parental expectations ("overstimulation"); difficulties precipitated by cross-cultural misunderstandings; and moves of school where the change for the child has been a radical one, e.g. from some rural to urban school settings.

An important part of the assessment is contact with the school, by phone or preferably in person in order to obtain a detailed account of the child's problems. The school's approach to the problem and the relationship between the teacher, child and parents are vital "informal" areas that are seldom officially reported.

The co-morbid conditions that may be present are: attention deficit disorder, language disorder, oppositional disorder, conduct disorder, depression and anxiety. These should be inquired about. Children with language disorder have delayed development of speech, delayed sentence construction and abnormal word production and their understanding of language may very. Many also have behavioural problems.

EXAMINATION

As for other disorders, the child may be more attentive in the office setting than in the class, where there are potentially more distractions.

In all cases an assessment of vision and hearing and a neurological examination are necessary and occasionally an assessment to rule out sleep apnoea. The psycho-educational assessment will include: standard tests of intellectual level and "cognitive style"; standardised achievement tests; and tests that clarify areas of specific disability. At the time of such testing, children may become easily angry with themselves, anticipate failure and avoid the test or perhaps act as if they don't care about school or their parents' reactions.

MANAGEMENT

The school may be able to provide integration or special assistance in class. Case conferences between the school and the professional may be useful in arriving at a fuller understanding of the problem and more integrated solution to the learning and behavioural problems. Assessments and treatments include family and/or school based behavioural management, cognitive behavioural therapy, family therapy, social skills groups and cognitive, academic and neuropsychological assessment and rehabilitation.

37 The Limping Child

HISTORY

Injury is probably the commonest cause and may be either due to direct impact (fractures, bruises, sprains) or is penetrating (lacerations, thorns, splinters, foreign bodies). If the nature of injury does not correlate with clinical illness, child abuse should be suspected.

Infection: An irritable hip limp might follow a simple viral upper respiratory tract infection after some seven to ten days. This commonly presents by refusal to walk after waking in an otherwise well child. Infection (osteomyelitis, septic arthritis) may be acute in onset and accompanied with fever and systemic disturbance, whilst chronic infection may have resulted in septic dislocation of the hip, stiffness of hip or knee or shortening of the leg. Other joints may be involved in various infective or inflammatory polyarthropathies. In most cases the aetiology may be obvious, e.g. rheumatoid arthritis, arthritis following rubella immunisation.

Referred pain: Pain in the knee in a child or adolescent is due to hip disease unless proved otherwise. Pain in the hip and/or thigh may be referred from the lower spine, paraspinal areas, abdomen and inguinal area.

In a young boy with a swollen painful knee, a family history of bleeding problems suggests a hemarthrosis as the cause of the limp.

A history of fever, weight loss, malaise and fatigue suggests the presence of a systemic disease such as malignant bone tumours, leukemia, and autoimmune diseases.

PHYSICAL EXAMINATION

The child should be asked to walk, tiptoe, heel walk, tandem walk and if possible, to hop on each leg. In most instances the pattern of the limp will be obvious and well recognised.

Antalgic limps are marked by unequal cadence as the child hurries off the painful leg. Short leg limps will show pelvic tilt and possibly a short leg scoliosis. Shortening above the greater trochanter will be associated with a positive Trendelenburg sign. Trendelenburg sag is due to altered hip geometry or abductor weakness. It is seen in fractured neck of femur, slipped upper femoral epiphysis, dislocated hip, coxa vara or coxa breva and painful or paralytic hip conditions which cause weakness of abductors. Paralytic limps vary according to whether they are upper or lower motor neurone lesions and the extent of the neurological deficit.

Rhomberg's sign, the Trendelenburg sign and a careful assessment of pelvic symmetry, spinal alignment and mobility and a detailed neurological assessment are required.

The skin should be carefully inspected for redness, warmth, bruises or puncture wounds as they may indicate pathology involving the underlying subcutaneous tissue, muscle or bone.

Special attention should be paid to the range of movements in the major joints of the lower limb and to leg lengths, both apparent and real. Apparent shortening is due to fixed deformity. Pain with active but not passive movements suggests a muscle or tendon problem.

Conditions such as iridocyclitis, rheumatoid nodules, erythema nodosum, carditis, and neurocutaneous stigmata should be looked for during the general examination.

DIAGNOSIS AND MANAGEMENT

Injured children may require X-ray examination if fracture or dislocation is suspected. Ultrasound is the method of choice for imaging splinters and thorns.

Most soft tissue injuries respond to RICE (rest, ice, compression, elevation). Those with actual bony injury should be referred to a children's casualty department.

Infective disorders will show no radiological changes for 7–10 days. Ultrasound or bone scan examination [Figs. 37(a)–37(c)] are the more appropriate investigations for early diagnosis. Children with septic arthritis must have the joint aspirated, whilst those with osteomyelitis may be given a trial of intravenous antibiotics. Blood cultures must be undertaken prior to administration of antibiotics unless a bacteriological diagnosis has been made by aspiration.

Intravenous flucloxacillin and amoxycillin are recommended for initial therapy until microbiology suggests a change. Though *Staphylococcus aureus* and *Streptococcus pyogenes* are the common organisms at all ages, 30% of infections in children under the age of 4 years are due to *Haemophilus influenzae*.

There are a number of orthopaedic conditions in children presenting with limp that are age specific:

Under Three Years Old

Toddlers fracture: The only common accidental injury leg fracture seen in this age group will cause an antalgic limp or refusal to walk. X-rays commonly reveal no abnormality and occasionally a bone scan will be necessary.

Undiagnosed congenital dislocation of the hip: Unilateral are marked by a Trendelenburg lurch and if bilateral, by an attractive waddle.

Congenital short leg: Any focal deficiency or reduction defect may be to blame and hemihypertrophy or hemiatrophy can cause a limp at this age.

Three to Five Years

Kohlers disease: Avascular necrosis of the tarsal navicular causes a painful swollen foot and an antalgic limp. The reaction is sufficiently severe to be confused with acute osteomyelitis. X-rays will show fragmentation and collapse of the navicular. A brief period in plaster is required.

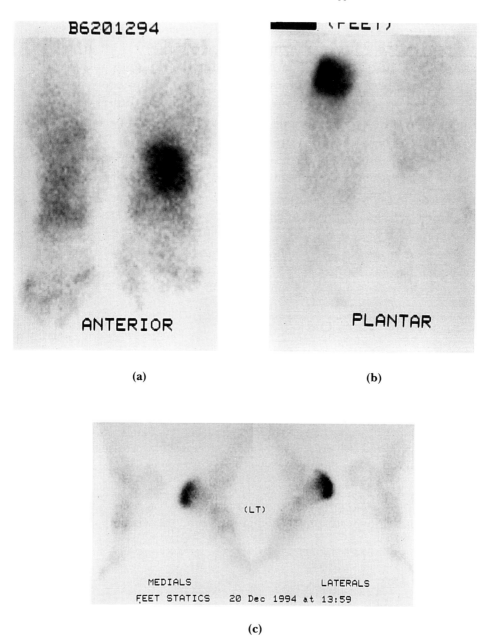

(a)   (b)

(c)

Figs. 37.1(a)–(c)   *Osteomyelitis of calcaneum.* Bone scans show increased uptake of radionuclide technetium.

Four to Nine Years

Perthes' disease: Usually presents as a gradually worsening limp. The limp may be antalgic, stiff hip, Trendelenburg or a combination of these types. Pain is not common in the early stage when X-rays may not reveal the condition, but a bone scan may show a void area if there is significant avascular change in the femoral head. These patients, most commonly boys, will always have restriction of abduction in flexion and internal rotation in extension. The problem is not an urgent one except for clarification and reassurance. Simple bed rest is the initial treatment required for the child with a bad limp or significant pain.

Eleven to Thirteen Years

Slipped upper femoral epiphysis: This condition occurs in pre-pubertal children, the majority of whom are overweight and have delayed secondary sexual development. Epiphysiolysis may be acute or gradual. Acute slips mimic fractures in their presentation. Gradual slips present with a painful limp. The pain is frequently referred to the knee or the thigh and less frequently experienced in the groin. Progressive external rotation of the affected leg may be noticed as the slip increases. Clinical examination will show restriction of abduction and internal rotation and frequently, increased external rotation. X-rays are required and a frog leg lateral is the best view to order, to ensure diagnosis. These patients require urgent treatment and assessment in hospital. Acute slip on top of a chronic slip can be a disaster as avascular necrosis is a common complication.

Ten to Sixteen Years

The osteochondritides: Activity-related disorders in rapidly growing children undertaking strenuous sporting or recreational pursuits may result in limping. Most of these are in fact pre-pubertal articular or epiphyseal cartilage injuries.

Osteochondritis dissecans: An osteochondral lesion of the femoral condyle which may cause knee pain. If a loose body forms it may produce severe mechanical symptoms. A tunnel view X-ray is usually diagnostic.

Osgood Schlatter's disease: is a traction apophysitis of the tibial tubercle. A swollen tender lump below the patellar ligament is diagnostic and X-rays are rarely needed to confirm the clinical picture. If acute, six weeks plaster cylinder immobilisation will often abort the problem and permit early return to moderate sporting activities.

Sever's disease: This is a traction apophysitis of the os calcis insertion of the Achilles tendon. When very painful, the children tend to walk on tiptoe to relieve the pull of this tendon. It is hurtful but not harmful. Relief comes by modifying activities, wearing higher heels or periods of immobilisation in plaster.

In most cases, the diagnosis of the cause of limp due to **neurological diseases** can be made from the history (including family history) and physical examination. Virological studies, cerebrospinal fluid examination, nerve conduction studies, muscle biopsy, serum creatine phosphate levels and imaging (CT scan, myelogram and MRI) may be necessary for aetiological diagnosis to offer definitive treatment and prognosis.

Patients with **systemic disease** require special investigations for diagnosis. ESR is raised in autoimmune, malignant and infective diseases. Full blood count and bone marrow aspiration will be required for patients suspected to have leukaemia and X-ray of the bone and bone biopsy are indicated for patients with suspected bone tumours.

38 Obesity in Childhood

Obesity is characterised by excessive deposition and storage of fat. The criteria for diagnosis require comparison of weight for age, weight for height and skin fold thickness. An accepted criteria is body weight exceeding expected norm for height by 35%. Irrespective of the underlying aetiology, obesity is always caused by caloric intake in excess of expenditure.

HISTORY

A dietary history is mandatory. In establishing accurate estimates of caloric intake, liquid food (orange juice, milk) should be listed separately. The child's frequency of food intake and the rationale for it should be elicited. Eating habits including, swallowing without chewing, gulping and source of food should be recorded. The supervision of eating and meals requires detailed analysis. Historical support for lack of satiety or over-stimulation of hunger centres should be sought. Careful diaries of daily physical activity and food intake have to be kept. All drugs should be listed and the possibility of their contribution to obesity should be considered. Height and weight data over time are crucial for determining the age of onset, chronicity and recent changes in velocity of weight gain. Family history of obesity, social history and an account of family interaction (including at meals) has to be ascertained.

PHYSICAL EXAMINATION

All previous and present height and weight measurements should be plotted carefully on growth charts. If the increase in weight has been continuous, endocrinological causes other than hyper-insulinism can be excluded. The distribution of adipose tissue will also help in arriving at a diagnosis. Truncal obesity is observed in Cushing's syndrome which is also accompanied with cessation of linear growth. Excessive adipose tissue in the sub-scapular region is seen in simple obesity which is associated with tall stature and precocious development.

General physical features of obese patients include a pendulous abdomen, white or purple striae on the abdomen, apparently small genitalia in boys as the penis is embedded in pubic fat, apparent breast hypertrophy and genu valgum.

Obesity may also be a presenting symptom of systemic diseases. Dysmorphic features, fundoscopic changes, subcutaneous calcification or retarded intellectual development should direct the differential diagnosis to genetic causes such as Prader Willi syndrome, Lawrence–Moon–Biedel syndrome and pseudo-hypoparathyroidism. Skin abnormalities such as acanthosis nigricans, pigmentation, colour and distribution of striae and hypertension will suggest specific syndromes such as insulin resistance, excessive glucocorticoid production. In these patients, a detailed neurological and developmental evaluation should be carried out. In the very obese child, an orthopaedic evaluation including testing for decreased muscle tone, slipped epiphyses and acquired abnormalities of knee and ankle joints has to be looked for.

MANAGEMENT

Most obese patients require few tests other than bone age, glucose-insulin ratio, serum electrolytes, haemoglobin and urinalysis for glucose and ketones. In endocrine causes of obesity, the bone age is retarded, whereas in simple obesity, the bone age is advanced. When specific syndromes are suspected, additional tests will be necessary.

Prevention is most important especially for those children at risk. Successful therapy of obesity requires a positive attitude and incentive on the part of the patient as well as the family. Unless the child is well motivated, it will be difficult to induce weight loss in the paediatric population. It is important to remember that in the paediatric population, successful treatment of obesity is already accomplished by maintaining a stable weight while growth continues.

Specific therapeutic suggestions have to be tailored for each individual patient. In some patients very significant reduction in caloric intake can be achieved by eliminating all liquid caloric intake. Concerned patients can be assured that vitamins and calcium, if required, can be taken in tablet form. Yet other children may respond by accepting a high residue, low calorie diet. All obese children however, require increased physical activity, not only in the form of a daily exercise programme, but also by walking, bicycling and limiting TV watching (to a maximum of 2 hours/ day). All obese children do need social interaction with peers and recreational outdoor activities.

Support has to be elicited from the entire family who have to accept that meals may have to be altered and that certain "junk foods" can no longer be stored in the house. Whenever possible, these children should not be left unsupervised, especially after returning from school. Most importantly, encouragement and praise have to replace nagging and scolding.

39 The Pale Child

Anaemia causing pallor is usually recognisable when the level of haemoglobin is below 8 g per 100 ml but at times vasoconstriction, dehydration and fair complexion may cause difficulties in interpretation.

HISTORY

1. *Duration of symptoms.* If of short duration, consider the possibilities of acute bleeding or haemolysis as contributing to the symptoms. If of longer duration (over one to two months), nutritional deficiency, marrow hypoplasia or infiltrative disease may be considered as possible aetiological factors.

2. *The age* of the infant or child. Under the age of six months, prematurity, bleeding, haemolysis and red cell hypoplasia are potential causes of anaemia. Between the ages of 7 and 18 months, iron deficiency is very common and in older children, marrow suppression, infiltrative diseases and chronic haemolytic disorders are more likely.

3. *Symptoms* may be variable, but give useful clues to the underlying disorders:

   - Fatigue usually indicates a more severe anaemia.
   - Dyspnoea may be due to severe anaemia and cardiac impairment or sometimes to a large intrathoracic mass, such as a mediastinal tumour, usually due to a lymphoma or leukaemia.
   - Appetite is often decreased in malignant disease or infections but in iron deficiency anaemia the infant usually may be drinking

140

abundant milk at the expense of solids.

- Limb pain and a limp may be due to infiltration such as leukaemia or neuroblastoma.
- Headaches may reflect severe anaemia or intracranial bleeding or infiltrative disease.
- Abdominal pain often is not well localised. It may be due to organ enlargement, especially with acute hepatosplenomegaly in leukaemia or to acute haemolysis or haemorrhage. Abdominal pain also occurs with sickling crises in sickle cell anaemia or in paroxysmal haemoglobinuria. In older children the pain may be more precisely localised, e.g. bone infiltration in leukaemia, lymphoma and neuroblastoma may produce localisation to the lower costal (rib) margins or the pelvis.
- Change in *urine colour* (red or "dark") may be due to haemorrhage (haematuria), or haemolysis, where the pigment may be due to urobilin or haemoglobin. Haemoglobinuria is indicative of intravascular haemolysis.
- Jaundice with anaemia usually indicates the presence of haemolysis.
- The colour of the stools may change and with haemolysis it often becomes darker.
- Associated bruising or bleeding is indicative of thrombo-cytopaenia, a qualitative platelet defect or coagulation disorder. Petechiae are usually associated with thrombocytopaenia.
- Lumps such as enlarged lymph nodes may be due to infection or infiltration.

4. Assessment of possible aetiological factors:

    (a) A *family history* of a similar disorder should be sought and some knowledge of the mode of inheritance is needed, e.g. autosomal recessive disorders include thalassaemia major, Fanconi's aplastic anaemia and some rarer hereditary red cell enzyme defects such as pyruvate kinase deficiency. Only the homozygotes will have the disease. Autosomal dominant disorders such as hereditary spherocytosis and von Willebrand's disease usually have a history of an affected parent.

    X-linked disorders such as haemophilia occur in males and red cell glucose-6-phosphate dehydrogenase (G-6-PD) deficiency usually occurs in males, but the double heterozygote female may also express the disease.

(b) *Antecedent illnesses.* Viral infections such as exanthemata, respiratory infections or EB virus are often implicated in the aetiology of immune thrombocytopaenic purpura and may be causal factors in autoimmune or cold antibody mediated haemolytic anaemias. Hepatitis may precede the onset of aplastic anaemia.

(c) *Chemical or drug exposure.* A history of such exposure should be sought especially in children with suspected marrow aplasia or cytopaenia. In G-6-PD deficiency, haemolysis may be attributable to broad beans, naphthalene, sulphonamides, antimalarials, while in marrow aplasia a history of administration of antimicrobials (chloramphenicol, sulphonamides), anti-rheumatic agents, antithyroid drugs and anticonvulsants in the previous six months should be sought.

(d) *Dietary factors.* A poor intake of iron with a very high milk and poor solid intake in the child aged 7 months to 2 years is fairly characteristic of iron deficiency. The infant of a vegan mother should be suspected of vitamin B_{12} deficiency if anaemia is associated with weakness, neurological deficiencies and slow development.

PHYSICAL EXAMINATION

General examination should include assessments whether the child looks sick, tired, pale, distressed or in pain and facial or body characteristics. A sick looking child may have an infection or malignancy. The centile charts should be consulted to assess the child's height, weight and head circumference. Small stature may be noted in thalassaemia major, Fanconi's anaemia and malabsorption syndromes. A relatively large head may be characteristic of a hyperplastic bone marrow as in chronic haemolytic anaemias and thalassaemia major. Particular facial and body features are detectable in Fanconi's anaemia, thalassaemia major, chronic haemolytic anaemias and hypothyroidism.

On closer inspection, jaundice, bruising, petechiae and obvious lumps should be sought. Physical anomalies may include those typical of Down syndrome or microcephaly, microphthalmia, skin pigmentation and cafe-au-lait spots, squint, hypoplastic or absent thumbs and radial deformities as noted in many children with Fanconi's anaemia. Joint swellings and a limp may be due to haemarthrosis, arthritis or associated with haematological malignancies. Enlargement of the liver, spleen or lymph nodes should be sought as well as evidence of masses in the abdomen or elsewhere. While a barely palpable spleen is often of no major clinical significance, a larger spleen exceeding 3 cm may be indicative of infection due to EB virus, toxoplasmosis, malaria, cytomegalovirus or other viruses or to haemolysis, infiltration or congestion with portal hypertension. Hepatosplenomegaly is more likely to be associated with leukaemia, thalassaemia major, some viral infections such as infectious mononucleosis and storage diseases. Splenomegaly alone is more consistent with haemolytic anaemias or congestive splenomegaly. Bone marrow hypoplasia is not associated with hepatomegaly or splenomegaly. In leukaemia, hepatosplenomegaly is commonly but not invariably present. Other abdominal masses, particularly if firm and non-tender, are likely to be due to a neoplastic process.

Excessive bruising is of greater importance if present on areas not usually subject to trauma, such as the hips, abdomen, chest and shoulder, implicating a platelet or coagulation defect. A haemarthrosis is usually due to a coagulopathy.

With a severe anaemia, especially of rapid onset, tachycardia, an ejection systolic murmur and wide pulse pressure may be found.

Examination of the chest should include a search for enlarged supraclavicular and axillary lymph nodes and checking for increased mediastinal dullness. Mediastinal masses and pleural effusions occur in non-Hodgkin's lymphoma.

Neurological examination should include the fundi for retinal haemorrhages or papilloedema, cranial nerves (facial or trigeminal nerve disorders may present in lymphoma or leukaemia) and the lower limbs for disordered gait. In neuroblastoma, lymphoma and rhabdomyosarcoma such gait disturbances sometimes associated with bowel or bladder dysfunction may herald impending paraparesis.

The mouth and the throat should be examined for evidence of ulceration or infection.

An outline for the diagnosis of the various types of anaemia in childhood is given in Tables 39.1 and 39.2.

Table 39.1   Clinical Diagnostic Possibilities in the Pale Child

---

A. PALLOR WITH ONE OR MORE OF THE
**   FOLLOWING   CONSIDER**

1. JAUNDICE   Haemolysis

2. HAEMORRHAGE   Coagulation disorder
                                Thrombocytopenia
                                Aplastic anaemia
                                Leukaemia

3. LYMPHADENOPATHY   Infection*
                                Leukaemia

4. HEPATOSPLENOMEGALY   Infection*
                                Leukaemia
                                Thalassaemia major

5. SPLENOMEGALY   Infection*
                                Haemolysis
                                Leukaemia
                                Portal hypertension with bleeding

B. PALLOR WITHOUT ABOVE
**   SIGNS AND SYMPTOMS**   Iron deficiency
                                Thalassaemia minor
                                Infiltration (leukaemia, non
                                Hodgkin's lymphoma,
                                neuroblastoma)
                                Lead poisoning
                                Inflammatory or chronic disease
                                Renal disease
                                Hypothyroidism
                                Aplastic anaemia
                                Megaloblastic anaemia
                                Haemolytic anaemia

---

* e.g. Epstein Barr virus, cytomegalovirus, toxoplasmosis

Table 39.2   Investigations likely to be helpful in the Diagnosis of Anaemias in Childhood

INVESTIGATION	HELPS IN DIAGNOSIS OF
1. BLOOD COUNT	
(a) Hypochromic red cells and microcytosis (MCV < 70fl)	Iron deficiency haemoglobinopathies, chronic blood loss and occasionally chronic infections.
(b) Macrocytosis (MCV > 95fl)	Megaloblastic anaemia, regeneration after blood loss, haemolysis or previous aplasia.
(c) Microcytosis with normochromia	Spherocytosis
(d) Anisocytosis and poikilocytosis	Consistent with dyserythropoiesis and haemolysis.
(e) Specific morphological red cell abnormalities	Haemolytic disorders (such as spherocytosis, crenated or burr cells, fragmented cells, blister cells and marked autoagglutination).
(f) Pancytopenia	Leukaemia, aplastic anaemia, megaloblastic anaemia, haemophagocytic syndrome and occasionally neuroblastoma.
(g) Reticulocyte count	Raised in haemolysis and regeneration, decreased in marrow hypoplasia or infection.
(h) Special blood film	Haemoglobin H disease, G-6-PD deficiency, sickle cell anaemia.

(e)   Antibiotics for associated bacterial infections.
(f)   Bone marrow transplant for aplastic anaemia, high risk leukaemia
      and some malignancies.

Symptomatic relief of discomfort or pain or bleeding may be required.
Paracetamol is the preferred analgesic initially.

Careful explanation of the nature of the illness, prognostic
implications and management should be given.

40 Polyuria and Polydipsia

Excessive production of urine (polyuria) is usually either due to the inability of the kidney to concentrate urine or due to high osmotic load in the urine. Polydipsia in these patients is secondary to the polyuria. Rarely polydipsia is due to compulsive water drinking which results in secondary polyuria.

HISTORY

The physician should ascertain whether the complaints are real or parental misinterpretation of symptoms. It should be established first, whether frequent urination or both urinary frequency and thirst are present and if so whether they are present during day and night (waking up at night to pass urine or drink water). In early infancy, the child cries excessively and will not be satisfied with additional milk but is quietened with water. There may be hyperthermia, rapid loss of weight or failure to grow. In older children, the presenting symptom may be bed wetting. Children with compulsive water drinking do not wake up at night to drink water and often insist on drinking tasteful fluids rather than water.

Other symptoms will depend on the underlying disease process, e.g. children with renal disease usually fail to thrive, those with diabetes mellitus give a history of recent loss of weight, those with tumours in the region of the hypothalamus may have disturbance of growth, progressive weight loss or obesity, hyperpyrexia and sexual precocity.

Family history of polyuria would suggest a diagnosis of diabetes insipidus (nephrogenic as well as pituitary) or diabetes mellitus.

EXAMINATION

The patient's weight, height and head circumference should be charted and compared with previous measurements. The patient's pulse rate, blood pressure and hydration will indicate the severity of fluid imbalance. Abnormal fundoscopic and visual findings would support a diagnosis of pituitary disease. Exophthalmus and pallor may be the prominent physical signs in patients with histocytosis X.

MANAGEMENT

An early morning urine sample after awakening with an osmolality of more than 600 mosm/kg excludes a diagnosis of diabetes insipidus. In such cases, urine should be examined for sugar and calcium and/or laboratory evidence of renal disease should be sought which would include urine analysis (albumin, microscopic examination and culture), serum and urinary electrolytes, creatinine and osmolality and 24 hour urine for volume, osmolality and creatinine.

Patients with low morning urine osmolality need further investigations to determine whether they have compulsive water drinking, renal or pituitary disease. Patients with compulsive water drinking are able to raise their urine osmolality after a period of fasting and those with pituitary disease will concentrate their urine following vasopressin given intra-nasally. Further investigations will be needed to determine the cause of renal or pituitary disease before instituting specific treatment. Long acting vasopressin preparations are contraindicated for infants.

Reassurance of parents and behaviour modifications will be successful in habitual polydipsic children (compulsive water drinking).

41 Rash

Rashes are very common in children and accompany many infectious diseases. A specific diagnosis may be made because of its characteristics. However many infections cause similar skin manifestations.

HISTORY

The physician should ask when and where the rash first appeared, how it progressed and whether there were accompanying signs and symptoms such as fever, upper respiratory tract illness and pruritus. A family history of a similar illness such as measles, scabies or eczema may be a clue to the diagnosis. A history of exposure to sunlight, drugs, allergens and infectious diseases should be obtained. Of specific interest are the nature and duration of any accompanying symptoms and an accurate description of the initial appearance and the evolution of the skin lesions and signs and symptoms.

EXAMINATION

When examining a patient with a rash, the physician should ensure that there is adequate, preferably natural light. The whole of the patient should be examined — it is not enough to look at a child's arm with a rolled up sleeve or the child's back with a lifted shirt tail. Besides inspection, the rash should be palpated and described as accurately as possible. The number (few, many, numerous); pattern (discreet, annular, localised, generalised, symmetric); distribution (face/scalp, palms/soles, truncal, intertriginous, extremities, acral/perineum, extensor, flexor, mucosal); size; spread (centripetal, centrifugal, caudal); and other characteristics (present in exposed areas only which suggests photosensitivity, pruritus, scaling, crusting) of the lesions should be noted. In addition the colour (erythema, hypo- or hyper-pigmentation), blanching or non-blanching and the type of the lesions (macules, papules, vesicles, bullae, pustules, plaques or nodules, haemorrhagic) should be noted.

MANAGEMENT

The diagnosis of infectious diseases with a rash can sometimes be made from the prodromal symptoms and pathognomonic signs, for example, Koplik's spots of measles. In many cases the clinician can deduce that the patient has a viral, bacterial or rickettsial infection and the exact diagnosis can only be made by appropriate cultures or serological tests. Table 41.1 lists the features of rashes of some of the common childhood conditions that present with a rash.

Other than bacterial, fungal and some viral infections, the treatment of many diseases presenting with a rash is symptomatic. Some patients may require topical treatment with corticosteroids. Above all, the physician should do no harm. Overuse of drugs such as topical corticosteroids and antibiotics should be avoided. General measures include avoidance of allergens, avoiding sunlight in photosensitivity, wearing cotton clothing next to the skin, maintaining short and smooth finger nails, wearing adequate clothing to protect patients with itching, use of moistened gauze (wrapped around weeping areas to reduce oozing, emollients for dry skin to reduce itching and powders for moist or oozing surfaces to prevent maceration. Patients with severe itching may require oral antihistamines and topical antipruritic medications.

Table 41.1 Common Conditions with Rashes

1. Maculo-papular rashes

DISORDER	DISTINGUISHING FEATURES
Rubeola (measles)	Prodromal fever, rhinorrhoea, cough, conjunctivitis, Koplik spots; blotchy rash first appears on head and spreads to the trunk, arms and legs.
Rubella (German measles)	Posterior auricular and occipital lymphadenopathy; rash begins on face and spreads to body.
Roseola infantum	3–4 days high fever followed by fine maculo-papular rash beginning on the trunk and spreading to extremities; fades in 24 hours.
Erythema infectiosum (Fifth disease)	Begins with erythematous cheeks ("slapped cheek" appearance) followed by an erythematous symmetric maculo-papular rash on trunk. Lasts more than a week and appears lacy and reticulated when fading.
Infectious mononucleosis	Pleomorphic rash occurs in 5–15% of cases with fever, pharyngitis, lymphadenopathy and hepatosplenomegaly.
Enteroviruses (coxsackie viruses A2, 4,9,16,B13 & echo virus 9)	Fever with rash indistinguishable from rubella. More common in children aged less than 5 years.
Scarlet fever	Punctate or finely papular red rash appears first in flexural creases and

	spreads rapidly; pharyngitis and characteristic (strawberry) tongue.
Kawasaki disease	Prodromal fever, conjunctivitis, oral ulceration with polymorphic erythematous rash leading to desquamation; coronary artery aneuryisms.
Erythema marginatum	Begins as slightly red raised non-pruritic macules but extend outward to form wavy lines or rings with sharp margins; occurs mainly over the trunk and inner surfaces of arms and legs and is characteristic of rheumatic fever.
Erythema toxicum	Papules with punctum; may coalesce (Fig. 41.1).

2. Vesicular & Bullous rashes

Varicella	Lesions appear in crops; spread is centrifugal.
Herpes zoster	Limited to dermatomes, do not cross mid-line, may be painful.
Hand, foot and mouth disease (coxsackie viruses A16, A5 & A10)	Oral ulceration, maculo-papular rash on hands and feet rapidly becomes vesicular; may involve nappy area.
Rhus dermatitis	Caused by plants such as poison ivy, oak; linear streaks of vesicles at point of contact.
Epidermolysis bullosa	Appears as blisters with minor trauma.

Bullous impetigo	Superficial pustular eruption (Figs. 41.2 and 41.3).
Herpes simplex (Fig. 41.4).	Vesicles occur at mucocutaneous junctions, coalesce and scab
Molluscum contagiosum	Discreet pearly dome shaped papules with central umbilication; seen on face, eyelids, neck, thighs, fingers (Fig. 41.5).
Pustular melanosis	Seen at birth as small dry vesicles on a pigmented brown macular base.

3. Purpuric rashes

Meningococcaemia	Rapidly developing petechiae and ecchymosis in a febrile sick child.
Henoch-Schonlein purpura	Has characteristic distribution on buttocks, back of thighs and legs, dorsum of feet; may be maculo-papular or vesicular; may be accompanied with arthralgia, abdominal pain, oedema or haematuria (Fig. 41.6).
Thrombocytopenia	Petechiae and ecchymosis with or without minor trauma.

4. Pruritic rashes

Atopic dermatitis (eczema)	Is accompanied with erythema, papules, vesicles, oozing and crusting involving the cheeks, forehead and extensor surfaces of the extremities in infants; in childhood, flexor rather than extensor services are involved and skin thickening by lichenification is common.

Insect bites	Lesions may be maculo-papular or bullous; in scabies, linear burrows on wrists, ankles and web spaces of fingers and toes (Fig. 41.7).
Urticaria (hives)	Characterised by raised erythematous lesions with well circumscribed serpiginous borders and large wheals; may be associated with dermatographia.

5. Papular squamous rashes

Psoriasis	Red plaques with sharply demarcated irregular borders with thick silvery or yellowish scales; occur most commonly on scalp, knees, elbows, genitalia and umbilicus; nails may be involved.
Pityriasis rubra pilaris	Red horny papules surrounding hair follicles; palms and soles are red, thickened and fissured.
Pityriasis rosea	An initial red annular lesion with a scaly border is followed by a generalised rash; may be urticarial or vesicular (Fig. 41.8).
Lichen planus	Multiple polygonal flat top violaceous lesions (1–2 mm in diameter) that coalesce; appear on flexor surfaces.

6. Miscellaneous rashes

Photosensitive rashes	The rash resembles exaggerated sunburn but may be urticarial or bullous and results in hyper-pigmentation. May be caused by systemic drugs (tetracycline, sulphonomides, phenothiazines, chlorthiazides), topical agents (coal tar, plants, soaps, perfume, oils), errors of metabolism (porphyria, pellagra),

genetic disorders (xeroderma pigmentosa), disorders involving immune mechanisms (systemic lupus erythematosis, dermatomyositis, scleroderma), infectious diseases (recurrent herpes simplex infection), exacerbation of skin diseases (lichen planus, psoriasis, sarcoid, atopic dermatitis).

Erythema multiforme

The lesions are symmetrical, appear in crops, more common on the extensor surfaces; they may be macular, papular, nodular, urticarial or haemorrhagic. The disorder is regarded as a hyper-sensitive reaction due to drugs, infections and exposure to toxic substances.

Erythema nodosum

Painful, indurated, shiny, red, hot, elevated, ovoid nodules 1–3cm in diameter; occur most frequently symmetrically over the shins; found in association with tuberculosis, streptococcal and yersinia infections, histoplasmosis, oral drugs and collagen diseases (systemic lupus erythematosis, regional enteritis and ulcerative colitis).

Ring worm

May occur on scalp resulting in alopecia. On the body, dry mildly erythematous elevated scaly papules or plaque spread centrifugally while clearing centrally (Fig. 41.9).

Seborrheic dermatitis

Rash is dry, scaly, papular, erythematous, crusty; involves face, neck and nappy area; appears as cradle cap on scalp; superinfection with candida and *Staph. aureus* is common (Fig. 41.10).

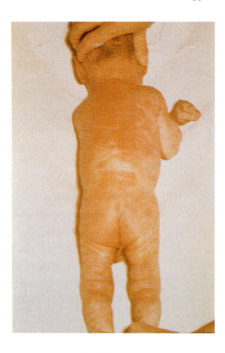

Fig. 41.1 *Erythema Toxicum.* The lesions on this infant have coalesced.

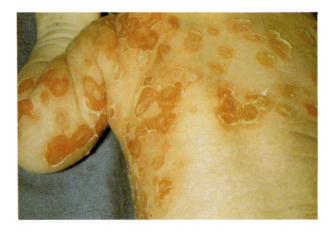

Fig. 41.2 *Staphylococcal bullous impetigo.*

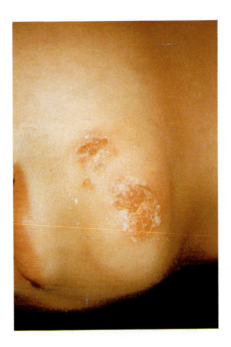

Fig. 41.3 *Streptococcus impetigo.*

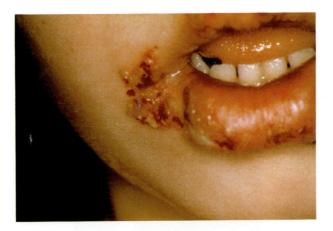

Fig. 41.4 *Herpes simplex.* Lesions consists of vesicles which coalesce and scab. Particularly occur at mucocutaneous junctions.

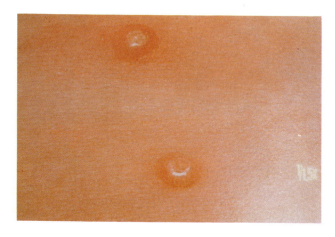

Fig. 41.5 *Molluscum Contagiosum.* Note the discrete pearly dome-shaped papules with central umbilication.

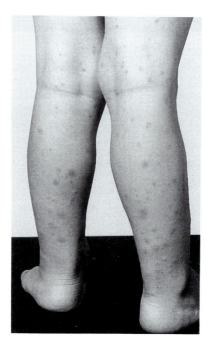

Fig. 41.6 *Henoch Schonlein Purpura.* The lesions (usually purpuric) are typically present on the buttocks and posterior aspects of the legs. This child also had joint pains.

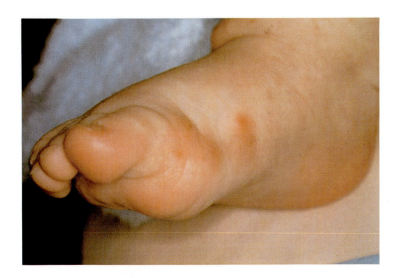

Fig. 41.7 *Scabies* with super-added infection due to scratching.

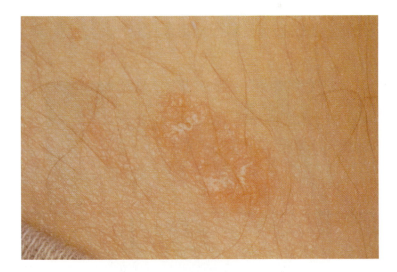

Fig. 41.8 *Pityriasis Rosea*. This initial scaly erythematous lesion is followed by a generalised rash.

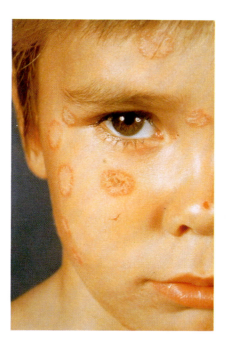

Fig. 41.9 *Tinea corporis.* The lesion is erythematous, raised, annular and scaly.

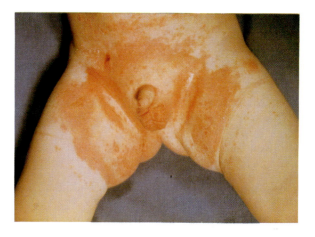

Fig. 41.10 Nappy rash with *Candida Infection.* Note satellite lesions.

42 Upper Respiratory Tract Infections

This section deals with structures of the respiratory tract above the larynx, namely nose, pharynx and ears. However, most respiratory illnesses affect both the upper and lower portions of the respiratory tract simultaneously or sequentially. Upper respiratory tract infections are more severe in infants and young children than in older children.

HISTORY

Children below the age of 3 months are afebrile. Those between the age of 3 months and 3 years have fever, irritability, restlessness and sneezing. The fever may appear a few hours before nasal discharge which may lead to nasal obstruction and moderate respiratory distress resulting in feeding difficulties. Some infants may vomit and have diarrhoea.

Older children have low grade fevers. Other symptoms are dryness and irritation in the nose and pharynx. These are followed by sneezing, chilly sensations, muscular aches, nasal discharge and sometimes coughing. Headache, malaise and anorexia may be present.

EXAMINATION

Nasal discharge is the prominent finding. Its consistency and volume will depend upon the stage of illness. Earlier it is thin, but later it may be purulent. There may be mucoid crusting and/or evidence of nasal obstruction (mouth breathing) which can cause moderate respiratory difficulty. The ear drums may be congested and fluid may be noted behind the drums.

MANAGEMENT

Many systemic infectious diseases (measles, rubella, pertussis, poliomyelitis, mumps, hepatitis, diphtheria) in their initial stage present with nasal discharge and have to be considered in the differential diagnosis. Allergic rhinitis is not accompanied by fever but there may be persistent sneezing and itching of the eyes and nose. Drug abuse, especially cocaine and marijuana should be considered in older children and adolescents with rhinitis.

Presence of unilateral, foul or bloodstained nasal discharge suggests the presence of foreign body or diphtheria.

In most cases the naso-pharyngitis is due to a viral infection and therefore antibiotics are of little value. Fever should be treated with paracetamol, but not with acetylsalicylic acid (aspirin) as the latter has been implicated in the causation of Reye syndrome. Nasal decongestants may be used if a child has difficulty with feeding, but otherwise their use should be minimal, as reactive hyperaemia and nasal obstruction will occur. Antihistamines do not alter the course of the disease and will only cause drowsiness in infants. Orally administered decongestants, though widely used, have not been shown to be of major value.

Nasal obstruction in infants may cause feeding problems. Suction with a soft-bulb syringe is occasionally helpful. Humidifiers and vaporisers may be useful in preventing drying of secretions.

43 Seizures in Childhood

HISTORY

Seizures are common problems in childhood. Because of the therapeutic and prognostic implications it is important to obtain a description of the type of fits, associated features, age of onset and to recognise the clinical symptoms and any possible aetiological factors.

1. The types of *seizure* based on the classification of the International League Against Epilepsy (ILAE) include the following descriptions:

   ### I. PARTIAL SEIZURES

   A. *Simple Partial Seizures*

   The discharge commences in one part of the brain and consciousness is not lost.

   1. With motor signs, these were previously referred to as Jacksonian seizures or focal motor seizures. Clonic seizure activity may start in a single muscle group from where it spreads to contiguous groups until an entire side of the body is involved. These seizures are often due to focal lesions located in the motor cortex in which the first affected movement originates.
   2. With peripheral sensory or special sensory (visual, auditory, olfactory, vertiginous) symptoms: the patient may have transient sensation of pins and needles or of numbness on one side. Sometimes there may be a focal onset as with the Jacksonian seizures. The focus lies in the sensory rather than motor cortex. Visual symptoms due to occipital lobe involvement or olfactory symptoms due to temporal lobe

involvement may be the presenting symptoms prior to the generalised convulsion.

3. With autonomic symptoms or signs: these include symptoms and signs such as pallor, flushing, headache, tachycardia, dilation of the pupils, abdominal pain and loss of bladder control prior to the onset of a seizure. In children, abdominal pain or enuresis may be the only symptoms.

B. *Complex Partial Seizures*

The discharge commences in one part of the brain but spreads to other parts resulting in alteration in consciousness. They have been referred to previously as pyschomotor or temporal lobe seizures. The early part of the attack is often remembered. Symptoms include hallucinations (visual, auditory) and sensation that an event had occurred previously (deja vu).

II. GENERALISED SEIZURES

A. *Absence Seizures*

1. **Typical:** Previously referred to as petit mal epilepsy. There is interruption of activities and staring or unresponsiveness of 5 to 15 seconds. Upward deviation of the eyes or rapid blinking may occasionally be present. Postural tone is not affected and there is no remembrance of the attack.

2. **Atypical:** These may have associated motor automatisms (such as lip smacking) or autonomic disturbances (e.g. loss of bladder control). At times, typical absence attacks become almost continuous over periods of hours or days in which case the child lapses into stupor.

B. *Myoclonic Seizures*: These are characterised by sudden muscle contraction (as in infantile spasms). In older children they result in sudden falls.

C. *Atonic Seizures*: These have been referred to as akinetic seizures or drop attacks. There is sudden relaxation of muscle tone and may be associated with falling, but with no loss of consciousness.

D. *Tonic-Clonic Seizures*: These are the most dramatic type of seizures. An attack may be preceded by an aura. The patient loses consciousness. Initially there is tonic contraction of the muscles followed by clonic movements. Respiration may be impaired. There may be involvement of the autonomic nervous system (excessive salivation, vomiting, and loss of bladder and bowel control). After the convulsion, the patient goes into a sleep-like state. In *status epilepticus* repeated tonic-clonic seizures occur without intervening recovery of consciousness.

The patient may have a *mixture of seizure types* which include atonic states, absences, myoclonic jerks or generalised tonic-clonic seizures as in the Lennox-Gestaut syndrome.

2. Associated features may include:

   (a) *Fever*: brief generalised convulsions associated with fever between the age of 6 months and 5 years in the absence of infection of central nervous system are typical *febrile convulsions*. Family history is often positive.

   (b) *Loss of consciousness*: is typical of grand mal seizures but is not always present with focal seizures.

   (c) Sensory rather than motor components or automatisms: occur with partial seizures.

   (d) *Hypoglycaemia*: an antecedent history of malaise for half-to-one day and *omission of several meals* may be found in children in seizures associated with hypoglycaemia.

   (e) *Breath holding attacks*: emotional or physical trauma is followed by cyanosis. The child may become unconscious and fall to the ground. Twitching may occur.

   (f) The *frequency of fits* may vary from occasional to many times a day. Seizures due to idiopathic epilepsy or Rolandic seizures may occur occasionally, while petit mal episodes, infantile spasms and Lennox-Gestaut seizures may occur up to hundreds of times in a day.

3. Seizure patterns and the aetiology of the seizure differ with age:

   (a) In the *neonatal period* fits are often atypical and include tonic, multifocal, focal and myoclonic fits. The seizures may be subtle and have to be distinguished from jitteriness and cyanotic attacks associated with apnoea. Subtle seizures **may** present as eye movements (deviation, blinking), sucking, **swimming** or pedalling limb movements or apnoeic episodes. Causes include hypoxia, ischaemia, intracranial haemorrhage, metabolic disturbances (hypoglycaemia, hypocalcemia, hypomagnesemia, inborn errors of metabolism), bacterial and viral intracranial infection and malformations of the brain.

(b) *In infancy*, after the age of 6 months and up to the age of 5 years, *febrile convulsions* are common. These comprise brief tonic-clonic seizures lasting less than 15 minutes with rapid recovery of consciousness and without localising neurological features and are associated with a fever usually over 38°C and without a primary neurological cause for the fever. Common causes are viral upper respiratory tract infections. The seizures may recur but the outcome is benign. In most instances the seizure has subsided by the time the child sees the doctor. Less common and much more serious are *infantile spasms* (West syndrome) occurring especially between 3 and 12 months of age. They are characterised by sudden flexor, extensor or mixed flexor-extensor muscle contractions of the neck, trunk or extremities, lasting only a few seconds but often in clusters many times a day. Aetiological factors are similar to those for neonatal seizures as well as tuberous sclerosis which account for 25% of such infants. *Breath holding attacks* can also cause seizures in this age group.

(c) *In early childhood* (3–5 years) idiopathic tonic-clonic seizures may occur. The Lennox-Gestaut syndrome appears at this age and is characterised by a variable group of seizure disorders with a mixed pattern such as brief but often frequent myoclonic, atypical absence and atonic generalised seizures. Several hundred episodes may occur in a day and children may fall during a seizure. The disorder is progressive and associated with developmental arrest. A past history of other forms of seizures (such as infantile spasms) or developmental delay may be present.

(d) *At school age* (more than 5 years of age), petit mal (childhood absence epilepsy), idiopathic or secondary partial seizures often occur. *Petit mal* attacks are characterised by brief absences and staring for about 10–15 seconds and can be confused with day dreaming. Falling does not occur. Attacks may be precipitated by over breathing. Many episodes may occur in a day. In the majority, attacks cease at or after adolescence. Atypical absences last longer than 30 seconds and are associated with disturbances of consciousness and often other movements. *Partial* or *focal seizures* may be motor (as in Jacksonian fits), sensory, (visual or auditory hallucinations) or complex associated with disturbed consciousness. The complex seizures may have aura (auditory, olfactory or visual) and unusual experiences such as deja vu (familiar previous experience), staring and automatisms followed by amnesia. Causes include perinatal illnesses, head injury, encephalitis, tumours and brain scarring. A type of benign partial epilepsy, or *Rolandic epilepsy* has an onset usually at 5–8 years, which is characterised by onset during sleep, awakening with one side of the face twitching and sometimes with gurgling sounds, lasting for less than two minutes. The frequency of episodes is low.

MANAGEMENT

The management of a seizure disorder may be divided into (a) management of an acute attack; (b) an aetiological diagnosis; and (c) long term management.

The first aim in the management of an acute attack is to stabilise the airway, breathing and circulation. Intravenous glucose (0.5–1 g/kg) may be useful in cases suspected of having hypoglycaemia. Intravenous diazepam (0.2–0.3 mg/kg) is indicated if the convulsions are persistent (diazepam can be given rectally if intravenous access cannot be achieved).

An aetiological diagnosis can be made by careful consideration of the history, physical examination and selective laboratory studies. Detailed information should be obtained about the characteristics of the seizure, other neurological or systemic disease and whether these are static or progressive in nature, past history including details of birth, post-natal course, development, serious illnesses, trauma, ingestions and toxic exposures, school performance and a relevant family history.

All patients should have a thorough neurological examination. In addition, the patient should be examined for the presence or absence of head bruits, skin lesions suggesting neurocutaneous disorders (cafe au lait spots, hypopigmented areas or haemangiomas; see Fig. 43.1) and cranio-facial or other skeletal deformities. It is useful to have a child hyperventilate in an attempt to provoke an attack. The history and physical examination should help the physician to distinguish between true seizure disorders and conditions such as breath holding spells, syncope, migraine, and benign movement disorders such as chorea.

The history and physical examination will establish a diagnosis in the majority of patients or help in planning further investigations. In patients with no definite diagnosis and many forms of epilepsy, the EEG is very useful in planning further management. Radiological studies such as CT scan and MRI may be necessary for an aetiological diagnosis.

Most seizures are self limiting and do not require emergency treatment other than ensuring that the patient does not hurt himself or has respiratory obstruction during an attack. Patients with tonic-clonic seizures may require intravenous anti-convulsant therapy (e.g. diazepam) to control the seizure. Prior to drug injection, a sample of blood should be withdrawn for measurement of glucose, calcium and electrolytes.

Long term anti-convulsant therapy will depend on the type of seizure and response to treatment.

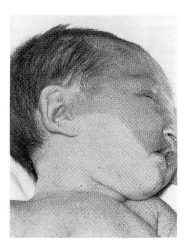

Fig. 43.1 *Sturge Weber syndrome.* The port wine stain on the face is associated with meningeal angioma which leads to cortical atrophy, seizures, mental retardation and contralateral hemiparesis.

44 Short Stature

HISTORY

Before the age of 2 years, few children will present with a history of short stature. In most cases the condition will be recognised on routine physical examination or may be part of some other disease process. It is most commonly due to failure to thrive (poor nutrition, chronic infections, congenital abnormalities) when the main problem is poor weight gain. Emotional disturbance, termed psychosocial dwarfism, can manifest as growth failure and short stature. Such infants have abnormal patterns of behaviour and may show signs of neglect or abuse. Various skeletal dysplasias may present as short stature or skeletal problems. Endocrine causes for short stature are almost always associated with preserved or even excessive weight relative to height. Associated symptoms may include constipation, poor feeding, lethargy (thyroid dysfunction) or mid-facial hypoplasia and micropenis with or without cryptorchidism (pituitary disorder).

Short stature associated with congenital growth hormone deficiency or congenital hypopituitarism usually does not become evident until the second 6 months of life or later. This diagnosis should be considered in any infant with a history suggestive of hypoglycaemia, particularly if there is also a history of neonatal jaundice.

In hypercortisolism (whether endogenous or iatrogenic), growth failure is one of the earliest signs.

PHYSICAL EXAMINATION

The weight, height and head circumference should be plotted on centile charts to determine the pattern of growth from birth. Plotting the height centiles of both parents will give the range of centiles within which the child should be growing. A mathematical method of assessment is to calculate the mid-parental height (see below). Besides the total height, the upper and lower segments should be measured. Particular attention should be paid to the examination of the skeletal system in order to diagnose congenital (chondrodystrophies) or acquired (rickets) diseases. Other signs will depend on the underlying disease process.

DIAGNOSIS

None of the pathological causes of short stature is age specific. In infancy, a length less than the third centile is most often associated with a similarly poor weight. Proportionately low length, weight and head circumference is suggestive of intrauterine growth retardation. Such patients may have stigmata of intrauterine infections or dysmorphic features that might indicate a congenital syndrome or chromosomal abnormality. In any girl with short stature, Turner's syndrome should be considered as short stature may be the only sign (Fig. 44.1). However, there may be a history of puffy hands and feet in the neonatal period and frequent ear infections in infancy and childhood. Other features include lower hair line, narrow fingernails, multiple naevi, neck webbing, shield-like chest and increased carrying angle of the elbow.

Skeletal dysplasia may be obvious morphologically (e.g. achondroplastic dwarfism). The diagnosis may be suggested by disproportionate growth of limbs or trunk which is evident on determination of body proportions (normally the upper to lower segment ratio decreases from approximately 1.7 at birth to 1 at puberty). See Figs. 44.2 and 44.3.

In order to confirm the diagnosis of growth hormone deficiency in infancy, it is necessary to demonstrate low levels (less than 2 ng/ml) of growth hormone on several occasions. In older children, especially over 5 years of age, a single estimation of somatomedin C is useful. In patients suspected of thyroid disease T3, T4 and TSH need to be measured. The bone age usually is delayed in growth failure due to endocrine causes but is not particularly helpful in differentiating between different causes of growth failure.

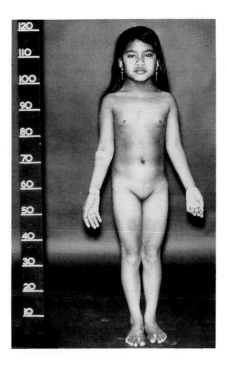

Fig. 44.1 *Turner syndrome.* Note short stature, webbing of neck and increased carrying angle. Karyotype 45X0.

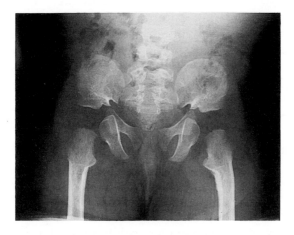

Fig. 44.2 *Achondroplasia.* X-ray shows sharply angled sciatic notches giving champagne glass appearance to pelvic inlet. Acetabular roofs are flat.

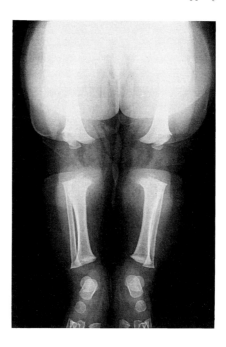

Fig. 44.3 *Achondroplasia.* Note short femoral shafts and broad short diaphysis with widened metaphysis.

Children with familial short stature grow at a normal rate (i.e. following a line below but parallel to the 3rd percentile) and are otherwise normal on history and physical examination. Sometimes there is an association of familial short stature with constitutional delay. In these cases, growth failure usually occurs in the first 5 years of life. There is often a family history of a similar growth failure or at least of delayed onset of puberty and a late growth spurt.

Mid parental height (in cms) is calculated as follows:

For a male = (father's height + mother's height + 13) ÷ 2

For a female = (father's height + mother's height − 13) ÷ 2

This mid parental height ± 5cm, marked on the prepared percentile chart, gives a range of percentiles within which the child should be growing.

45 Tall Stature

HISTORY

Just as short stature at any age is most likely to be familial, so is tall stature — hence the importance of knowing parental height in the assessment of tall stature. Isolated tall stature is an uncommon complaint in infancy and early childhood. Most of the patients are young girls whose parents are worried about the ultimate height.

In infancy and childhood, the obese child may be relatively tall for the family background. Body proportions will be appropriate for height age. There are several syndromes of overgrowth in infancy and childhood (e.g. Sotos' syndrome, Weaver's syndrome and Beckwith-Wiedemann syndrome). The diagnosis is suggested by other abnormal physical findings corresponding to the pattern of dysmorphism specific for each syndrome.

Tall stature in the prepubertal age group may be associated with accelerated growth due to excess steroids of gonadal or adrenal origin. Such children may present with oily skin, acne, body odour, pubic or axillary hair growth, enlargement of the penis or clitoris, breast development, vaginal discharge or testicular enlargement.

Patients with Marfan's syndrome may present with joint laxity, visual disturbances and cardiac symptoms. Developmental retardation may be the presenting symptom of homocystinuria and other overgrowth syndromes.

PHYSICAL EXAMINATION

Physical findings will depend on the underlying aetiology. In all patients, previous weight and height measurements should be obtained.

Developmental retardation may be present in several syndromes of overgrowth in infancy such as homocystinuria, sex chromosome aneuploidy with excess X chromosomes (XXY, XXXY, XXXXY). In patients with excess steroid of gonadal or adrenal origin, there would be evidence of secondary sexual characteristics. Increased skin pigmentation especially in old scars suggests excessive ACTH secretion which is found in congenital adrenal hyperplasia. Genital abnormalities such as small phallus, hypospadius, and small testes will be found in boys with sex chromosome and aneuploidy with excess X chromosomes. During puberty, these boys develop gynecomastia and testicular growth is slow. Patients with tall stature due to a growth hormone producing pituiraty adenoma have large hands and feet with soft tissue overgrowth, coarse features, a prominent jaw and widely spaced teeth. Visual field defects may be present.

MANAGEMENT

In tall girls without underlying pathology, it is possible to predict the final height from the height and the bone age. It is possible to retard the ultimate height by administration of oestrogens but such treatment should not be undertaken without fully discussing with the parents and the patient the problems associated with oestrogen therapy.

In most cases the diagnosis may be obvious on physical examination and investigations are carried out to confirm it. Treatment is specific in conditions like homocystinuria, pituitary adenoma, adreno-genital syndrome but has to be symptomatic in the majority of cases.

46 Blood in the Stools

Although very frightening to parents, because of the association of blood with haemorrhage and with cancer, more often than not, blood in the stool of infants and young children is due to very benign causes.

HISTORY

It is important to distinguish between blood *on* or *in* the stool. Small amounts of blood *on* the stool in well infants and children most commonly result from an anal fissure associated with constipation. The stools may be streaked with blood or the blood may appear with discomfort at the end of defaecation. There is usually a past history of constipation. Haemorrhoids, although uncommon in children, can also present similarly but without the same degree of discomfort. Tiny streaks of blood *on* or *in* the stool are very common in young children but usually no cause is found.

Diarrhoea associated with blood, may be due to infection with organisms such as salmonella, shigella, yersinia, and campylobacter at any age. In early infancy, it may be a symptom of other forms of enterocolitis such as necrotising enterocolitis, cow's milk associated colitis, Hirschprung's enterocolitis and with older children with inflammatory bowel disease (ulcerative colitis or Crohn's disease), pseudo-membranous enterocolitis or antibiotic associated diarrhoea. When blood is associated with diarrhoea, the length of the history and the associated symptoms will usually give a very good indication of the underlying problem.

Old blood in the stool or melaena implies that the blood is coming from higher up in the bowel. Vomiting, acute colicky abdominal pain with passage of blood rectally in a child from 6 months to 3 years of age, suggests intussusception. On the other hand, painless passage of large amounts of blood in the same age group, may be associated with Meckel's diverticulum or duplication of the bowel. As intestinal polyps and bleeding diatheses can present with severe bleeding at any age, family history of polyps or blood dyscrasia should be sought, particularly if the bleeding is severe enough to produce anaemia or acute haemodynamic disturbance.

EXAMINATION

Unless the bleeding is severe, in most cases no abnormality will be found. In all patients, the anal area should be examined for excoriation and fissures. Anaemia may be present in patients with a severe or prolonged history of bleeding. Abdominal examination may reveal tenderness (inflammatory bowel disease), lumps (constipation, intussusception) or hepatosplenomegaly with dilated superficial abdominal veins (portal hypertension). In patients with blood dyscrasias, petechiae and ecchymosis may be found.

MANAGEMENT

Stool microscopy and culture are always indicated in such children looking for red and white blood cells and bacterial pathogens. The absence of leucocytes and pathogens implies bleeding without inflammation. Whether to proctoscope or endoscope such a child, then largely depends on the amount of bleeding, its chronicity and whether it is causing anaemia. Sometimes endoscopy may be necessary to allay parental fears but it is necessary to keep in perspective the invasiveness of the procedure and the bowel preparation required for it. Other investigations and treatment will depend on the diagnosis.

47 Strabismus

Strabismus occurs in approximately 3% of the population. Though familial tendency has been well documented, there is no clear cut genetic mode of inheritance. It may be congenital or acquired.

HISTORY

Strabismus may be present from birth. In most cases the parents or caregiver observes that it is only present when the child is tired. In other cases, it may become apparent following an acute illness. In many cases, a parent or another family member may give a history of strabismus in infancy. In older children, other symptoms may include visual disturbances (diplopia, myopia), headache and abnormalities of gait.

EXAMINATION

Rapid screening of strabismus is best carried out by the *corneal light reflection test*. This method has the disadvantage that there is a high incidence of false positive findings and the presence of a false negative result may give a false sense of security. The test is carried out by directing a pen light at the cornea and the observer notes the position of the corneal reflection with respect to the centre of the pupil. If the light reflex is deviated toward the nose, exo deviation is present; convergent deviation should be suspected when the light reflex is deviated towards the lateral side of the pupil (Figs. 47.1 and 47.2).

The *alternate cover test* is more sensitive for the detection of strabismus. It has the advantage that it results in a very low incidence of false

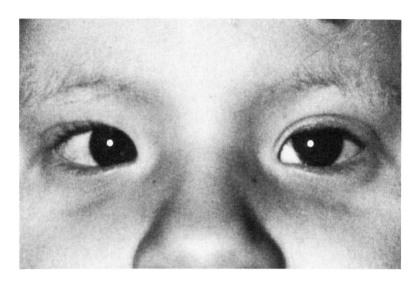

Fig. 47.1 *Pseudo-strabismus.* Note epicanthic fold on right. Corneal light reflection is identical in both eyes.

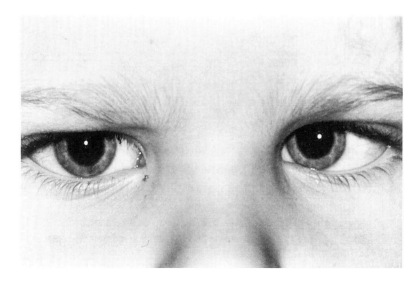

Fig. 47.2 *Convergent strabismus.* Note light reflection in the left eye is deviated towards the lateral side of the pupil.

negative findings. The test is performed by using a large object to attract the infant's attention and then alternately covering one eye and then the other with the hand or occluder. The presence of the shift of one eye while covering the other eye will occur if strabismus is present. Strabismus due to nerve palsy is diagnosed by testing for eye movements. A detailed neurological examination should be carried out in patients having strabismus due to nerve palsy.

Objection to covering one eye but not the other suggests the presence of amblyopia.

Incorrect diagnosis of strabismus can be made if the above two tests are not performed. This is particularly true in children who have epicanthic folds and broad flat nasal bridge. This is due to the decrease in the amount of nasal conjunctiva visible to the observer. The parent frequently reports that the eyes are crossed, more with the right or left gaze and with near viewing as convergence accentuates the illusion.

In all cases the eyes should be examined for local pathology and cranial nerve palsies. A detailed neurological examination is necessary as the strabismus may be the presenting sign of intracranial pathology.

MANAGEMENT

Up to the age of 2–3 months, normal infants can have intermittent strabismus. Persistence of strabismus beyond the age of 10–12 weeks needs further evaluation by an ophthalmologist. Treatment should be commenced as soon as possible but certainly before the age of 4 years as amblyopia is a complication of inappropriately managed strabismus.

Acquired strabismus requires further investigations as it may indicate underlying intracranial disease.

48 Stridor

Stridor is a harsh, medium pitched inspiratory sound that is caused by obstruction of the laryngeal area or the extra thoracic trachea.

HISTORY

The stridor may be recurrent or persistent. Persistent stridor may be present from birth or may appear soon after birth. Increase in stridor when a child is supine suggests laryngomalacia or tracheomalacia. Stridor with hoarseness or aphonia suggests involvement of the vocal cords.

If the stridor is persistent, it suggests a congenital abnormality causing narrowing of the laryngeal area or the extra thoracic trachea. These include laryngomalacia, papillomas, cysts, laryngeal webs, subglottic tracheal stenosis, mediastinal masses, vascular rings and thyroid enlargement in infants. Recurrent stridor occurs in allergic croup and respiratory infection in a child with anatomic narrowing of the large airways.

In well infants, acute stridor is usually due to viral croup and is accompanied with croupy cough and hoarse voice. In toddlers with a recent history of persistent stridor, information should be obtained about choking attacks as it may be due to a foreign body in the oesophagus or trachea. In children above the age of 2 years, acute stridor may be the presenting symptom of acute epiglottitis. Accompanying symptoms include fever, sore throat, drooling (as the child cannot swallow), hoarseness or aphonia, brassy cough, irritability, restlessness and prostration.

EXAMINATION

Patients with recurrent or persistent stridor due to congenital abnormalities do not have many physical signs. The patient may demonstrate mild suprasternal and subcostal recession and changes in severity and intensity of the stridor with changes of body position.

In viral croup, the physical signs will depend on its severity. In mild to moderate cases, there is nasal flaring, suprasternal and intercostal retraction and the child prefers to sit up in bed or be held upright. In severe cases, the physical signs are a result of hypoxia (restlessness, increase in pulse, dyspnoea) and decrease in air entry.

Patients with acute bacterial epiglottitis may have all the physical signs of acute croup. In addition they have sore throat, coarse inspiratory vibrations, tend to keep their mouth open with the tongue protruding and may rapidly progress to a shock-like state characterised by pallor, cyanosis and impaired consciousness. The diagnosis requires depressing the tongue to see the enlarged swollen cherry-red epiglottis. However, this should *not* be undertaken in a suspected case unless facilities for cardiorespiratory support are available as reflex laryngospasm, acute respiratory obstruction and cardiorespiratory arrest may follow examination of the pharynx.

MANAGEMENT

Patients with recurrent or persistent stridor require X-rays and airway screening to demonstrate localised narrowing of the trachea (Fig. 48.1). However, in most cases direct observation (endoscopy) is necessary for diagnosis.

In acute croup, the aim of treatment is to maintain adequate respiratory exchange. Steps should be taken to prevent agitation and crying as these greatly aggravate the symptoms and signs. Patients with mild croup and laryngeo-tracheo-bronchitis usually can be safely managed at home. They may respond to treatment with cold or hot steam, as these often terminate acute laryngeal spasm and respiratory distress within minutes. The same effect may also occur when the child is taken out into the cold night air on the way to the physician's office.

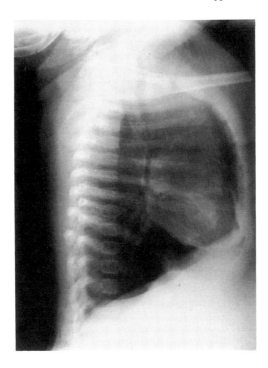

Fig. 48.1 *Vascular Ring* presenting as stridor. There is compression and deviation of the mid thoracic trachea.

In children with severe croup and high fever or other symptoms suggestive of epiglottitis, examination of the pharynx should be deferred until transfer to a hospital as cardiorespiratory arrest can occur following manipulation of pharynx (including use of a tongue depressor). As indicated earlier, examination of the pharynx should not be carried in patients suspected of having epiglottitis.

All patients with acute stridor due to croup or epiglottitis need close observation for symptoms of increasing respiratory obstruction by frequent or continuous monitoring of the respiratory rate, pulse rate, restlessness and colour. Regular adrenaline 1/1000 3 mls by aerosol may result in transient relief of symptoms in most cases and may prevent the need for nasotracheal intubation in severe cases. Sedatives and oxygen are contraindicated unless the obstruction has been relieved.

As epiglottitis is caused by *H influenzae*, these patients are treated with the appropriate antibiotics. The usual choice is ampicillin and chloromycetin or a cephalosporin. All contacts of the patient under the age of 5 years should be given prophylactic rifampicin.

Antibiotics do not have any place in the treatment of acute or recurrent croup or laryngo-tracheo-bronchitis. In severe cases, intravenous corticosteroids are recommended as they have been demonstrated to reduce the need for endotracheal intubation or tracheostomy.

49 Undescended Testes

HISTORY

The patient with undescended testis or testes may be identified on routine physical examination or may present to the doctor by the parents who found an empty scrotum. The age at which the problem is recognised is important as descent of the testis can occur up to the age of 1 year. Parents should be asked whether the condition is unilateral or bilateral, is intermittent or permanent, and if there are any other abnormalities of the genitalia. The physician should also inquire about the family history of undescended testis and infertility.

PHYSICAL EXAMINATION

During inspection, the examiner should note the development of the scrotum and the penis. Incomplete male genital development (hypospadias) suggests cryptorchidism to be a secondary event. On the other hand, simultaneous occurrence of cryptorchidism and micro-penis suggests abnormal sex hormone secretion in the latter half of pregnancy. When these findings are present, further investigations are necessary before surgical correction of the cryptorchidism.

During the examination, the child should be relaxed and the examiner's hands should be warm. The examiner should distinguish an undescended testis from a retractile testis. The scrotum in the latter case is usually rugose and normal. The testis can be found and brought to the bottom of the scrotum without difficulty where it stays upon release until stimulation. An undescended testis will usually be found somewhere along the line of normal descent and will be unable to be brought to the bottom of the scrotum. It usually stops at somewhere around the pubic tubercle or upper scrotal neck level. It is usually smaller and softer than the descended testis.

If a testis cannot be found in the line of descent, it may still be in the abdominal cavity, or it may have undergone complete atrophy due to torsion or it might lie in an ectopic position. The latter may be in the perineal, medial side of thigh or prepubic area and may be difficult to locate, but a cord can be felt in the inguinal canal and can be traced to the testis. A spermatic cord can be found in the inguinal canal in infants with atrophic testis.

MANAGEMENT

Patients with undescended testes and abnormalities of the penis should have chromosome analysis and radiological investigations in order to demonstrate or exclude the presence of female reproductive organs. In the first two days of life, the uterus is still firm and enlarged and is easily felt by rectal examination.

Retractile testes do not require an operation as they are normal testes which will come to lie permanently in the scrotum at puberty without any medical intervention. Medical therapy of undescended testis with chorionic gonadotropin (HCG), LHRH or testosterone will not be successful in true undescended testis unless due to LHRH or gonadotropin deficiency which is suggested by the presence of both micro-penis and undescended testis.

Testicular descent is still possible in the first year and so it is usual to defer an operation until 12 months of age. If a hernia should appear within the 12 months on the same side, then herniotomy and orchidopexy are performed at the same time as a semi-urgent operation. An operation should not be delayed beyond the age of 2–3 years as descent rarely occurs after that age and there is a risk of disturbance of testicular function.

If both testes are presumed to be intra-abdominal, gonadotrophin and testosterone level should be determined prior to operation. Elevated gonadotrophin levels are a contraindication to surgical exploration as they indicate the vanishing testes syndrome. In patients with other co-existing genital abnormalities, the karyotype should be determined prior to operation.

If a testis is impalpable, sometimes an ultrasound is performed, but it is very difficult to demonstrate a testis along the posterior abdominal wall, as bowel gas prevents visualisation. A testis within the inguinal canal is easily seen on ultrasound but should be able to be palpated. Surgical management of impalpable testis is to perform a groin exploration but it should not be undertaken without demonstrating normal gonadotrophin and testosterone levels. If the testis has undergone neonatal torsion, the vas and the vessels will be found in the inguinal canal and the remnant of the testicular tissue with a cord should be excised. It is important that the other testis be fixed to prevent its future torsion as the anatomical anomaly that caused the neonatal torsion is almost invariably bilateral, placing the other testis at risk. If no testis or cord is found in the inguinal canal, a retroperitonial exploration is performed and the undescended testis is brought down. Some surgeons perform a laparoscopy as a preliminary to locate a high intra-abdominal testis in order to facilitate the operation later. Testes that are too high should be brought down into the scrotum or excised as the risk of malignancy in such testes is very high. All undescended testes show abnormal morphology. As a result fertility with a unilateral undescended testis is between 60–90% of normal and with bilateral undescended testes, is 10% of normal. The onset of puberty is not affected.

50 Failure to Thrive

Thrive means to "flourish" or "grow". This term is used in paediatrics to identify infants and children who fail to gain weight and often lose weight without any obvious identifiable cause. The condition is most often seen in infants but may be observed in early childhood.

HISTORY

The history should aim to identify children who are small but otherwise normal (and hence require no further investigations) from those who have an ongoing pathological process. Low birth weight infants (both premature and small-for-dates) are usually small for their chronological age. Some of these children will have catch-up growth but others may remain small depending upon the aetiology. It is important to inquire about the weights and heights of parents and other siblings.

A careful dietary history is important as undernutrition is the commonest cause of failure to thrive. The undernutrition may be due to psychosocial deprivation or an underlying disease process. The history should aim to evaluate the caregiver's psychological status (depression) and attitude towards the child (neglect or abuse). Information should be obtained to determine whether the child has a physical handicap (cleft palate, cerebral palsy) which may prevent adequate food intake. In patients with adequate dietary intake, an attempt should be made to determine if there are excessive losses (diarrhoea, vomiting) or a catabolic state (chronic infection, history suggesting thyroid disease or diabetes or malignancy). Previous weights and height measurements should be obtained as these will indicate the time of onset of the problem.

PHYSICAL EXAMINATION

All the available data on the patient's weight, height and head circumference should be plotted on percentile charts to determine the pattern of growth. The patient's development should be assessed. Signs of physical and emotional deprivation such as apathy, poor hygiene, withdrawing behaviour, may be present. The aim of the physical examination is to exclude major abnormalities such as congenital heart disease, mental deficiency and pyschomotor retardation. In the majority of cases, no physical signs other than evidence of loss of weight (poor subcutaneous tissue, muscular wasting) will be found. Severe cases may show marasmus (Fig. 50.1) or kwashiorkar (Figs. 50.2 and 50.3).

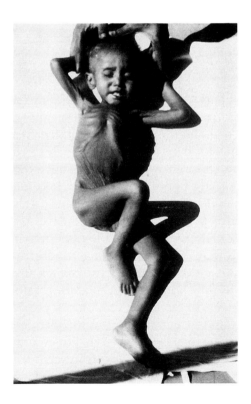

Fig. 50.1 *Marasmus.* Note extreme muscular wasting and loss of subcutaneous tissue.

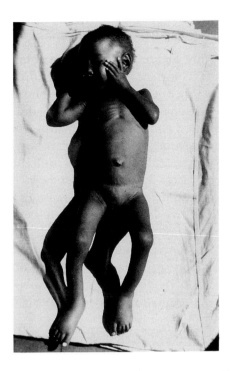

Fig. 50.2 *Kwashiorkar.* Note oedema of feet and everted umbilicus due to ascites.

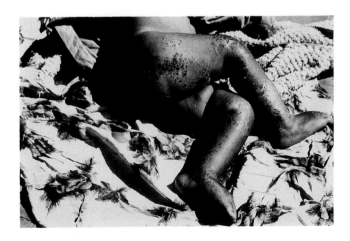

Fig. 50.3 *Kwashiorkar* showing hyper-pigmented hyperkeratotic skin lesions.

MANAGEMENT

The history may provide a clue to the diagnosis, but in the majority of cases the problem is complex. Hospitalising the child provides an opportunity for observing the child's correct intake and observing the interaction with the parents, health personnel and other children. In many cases, hospitalisation leads to dramatic improvement in weight gain which provides evidence that environmental factors are causative, thus eliminating the need for searching for other underlying organic disease.

If the history or physical examination suggests disturbance in any organ system, appropriate investigations may be carried out, e.g. sweat test or immunoglobulins in children with recurrent respiratory infections. In all cases, a few screening tests (full blood count, ESR and urine analysis) are appropriate but extensive investigations should be withheld until such time as a failure of a favourable response to hospitalisation has been demonstrated. A greatly reduced bone age compared to weight, height and chronological age will suggest an endocrine problem.

51 Sore Throat

Throat (and tonsillar) infections occur rarely alone and usually involve the adjacent structures. They can occur in various acute generalised infections, particularly diphtheria, herpangia, adenovirus infection and infectious mononucleosis. In this chapter, the condition which principally affects the throat, is described.

HISTORY

Acute pharyngitis rarely occurs before the age of 1 year. Incidence peaks at the age of 4–7 years though it continues throughout later childhood and adult life. Fever and sore throat are the principal symptoms. Unlike streptococcal infections, systemic symptoms (fever, headache, abdominal pain, vomiting) are less frequent with viral infections. On the other hand, nasal discharge is more common with viral infections. Other symptoms include cough and hoarseness of voice. The patient may present with bilateral cervical swellings due to enlargement of the lymph nodes.

EXAMINATION

Unlike viral infections, patients with streptococcal infection may appear toxic. The throat and tonsillar area appear erythematous. Petechial haemorrhages, small ulcers and exudates may appear on the soft palate, posterior pharyngeal wall, lymphoid follicles of palate and tonsils. The tonsils may be swollen and enlarged. The cervical lymph nodes may be enlarged and tender.

MANAGEMENT

It is impossible to distinguish viral from bacterial (mainly streptococcal) infections of the pharynx and tonsils clinically. White cell counts are of little value and the only method for diagnosis is by culture or in the case of streptococcal infections, by the demonstration of antigens.

The presence of a membranous exudate should alert the physician to the possibility of diphtheria or infectious mononucleosis. Patients with agranulocytosis may present with symptoms of acute pharyngitis — the diagnosis is usually made in retrospect when the result of the blood count is available.

As it is impossible to distinguish bacterial from viral pharyngitis or tonsillitis by clinical examination, antibiotic treatment should be guided by the results of antigen detection tests or cultures. In patients with proven streptococcal pharyngitis, penicillin should be administered for at least 10 days. Erythromycin may be used in patients with a history of allergy to penicillin.

There is no urgency to commence antibiotic therapy, even in a case of definite streptococcal infection, as complications such as rheumatic fever, acute nephritis do not occur unless the infection is not treated for at least a week. Therefore the routine use of antibiotics in all cases of acute pharyngitis is not justified.

In addition to specific treatment with antibiotics, symptomatic treatment of the fever with paracetamol is desirable in all cases. Gargles may be helpful in older children.

52 Severe Paediatric Trauma

In developed countries, injuries are the major cause of death in children aged 1 to 14 years and account for almost half the deaths from all causes in this age group. Road trauma and drowning account for more than 60% of the deaths due to accidents. The most frequently injured part of the body is the head followed by the chest, abdominal organs and cervical spine.

HISTORY

Usually this is obtained after assessment and emergency treatment of the child. However, it is important to obtain a careful history (whether the child was a pedestrian or a passenger in a car wearing a child restraint or not) which should include details of the mechanism of injuries and any treatment already given.

PHYSICAL EXAMINATION

It is not in the child's interest to seek a complete diagnosis until the adequacy of the airway, breathing and the circulation (ABCs) are ensured and a brief baseline neurological assessment is carried out. The cervical spine should be protected while the airway is assessed and managed, particularly in children who have an injury above the clavicle. The pulse rate, skin perfusion and blood pressure should be noted. The brief neurological assessment has two components only. Firstly the pupillary reaction and secondly the child's level of consciousness as determined by the commonly used mnemonic AVPU. The child is Awake or not awake but responding to Vocal stimuli or responding only to Painful stimuli or entirely Unresponsive.

Having identified and managed the immediately life threatening injuries, the child must be fully exposed so that all parts can be examined in order to identify all the injuries and particularly those that are not obvious. As heat loss in small children is a common problem, some form of external heating is recommended. If the wounds have already been covered, the dressings should be taken down so that the wounds can be properly assessed. Children can lose a significant proportion of their blood volume into the dressings before it is obvious.

The back and perineum are frequently forgotten and should be specifically examined, by log rolling the child to protect the spine.

MANAGEMENT

There are a number of specific factors that need to be considered when managing injured children. Being smaller than adults, children will have the same kinetic energy dissipated throughout their smaller body mass when involved in a similar collision, potentially causing more serious and more widespread organ injury. Occult injuries are common because of the pliable rib cage and the relatively underdeveloped abdominal musculature allows major damage to occur to underlying organs without external signs of injury. Their larger body surface area to body mass ratio allows for more rapid heat loss and this is a particular problem during resuscitation and operative intervention, especially with small infants. Their ability to maintain their blood pressure via vaso-constriction and tachycardia makes the blood pressure an excellent but very late indicator of hypovolaemia. Acute gastric dilatation is a common problem that can exacerbate other injuries and lead to diagnostic confusion. The psychosocial development of children can make their behaviour difficult to assess if the examiner is not used to dealing with sick children and the frequency of head injury will compound the problem.

The first step in efficient resuscitation is to recognise and manage the immediately life threatening problems (ABCs). Death or major morbidity will be most rapidly caused by airway obstruction, interference with breathing or an inadequate circulation. Even if an acute intracranial problem has developed, the initial management should be ensuring the adequacy of ABCs.

When assessing the circulation in an injured child, shock equals blood loss until proven otherwise. As described above, the blood pressure is an excellent late sign of hypovolaemia but the pulse rate, skin perfusion and urine output are the important early indicators. Hypovolaemia should be corrected by rapid infusion of colloid or crystalloid fluid bolus (20 mls per kg) followed by assessment of the patient's response. Further fluid (including blood products) should be titrated for the patient's need by ongoing reassessment. *It is important to remember that a normal blood pressure does not exclude shock and tachycardia is hypovolaemia and/or hypoxia until proven otherwise.*

If there is any deterioration in the level of consciousness then the first priority is the reassessment of the adequacy of airway, breathing and circulation (ABCs) as they may be the cause of the deterioration even in children with intracranial problems.

All children with multiple-trauma should have an X-ray examination of their cervical spine, chest and pelvis. Other X-rays should be performed as clinically indicated. Any "tube" that has been inserted (e.g. endotracheal, gastric or intercostal) should have its position confirmed on an X-ray before the child is transferred any significant distance. Blood should be taken for cross-matching, full blood count and electrolytes. Diagnostic peritoneal lavage, while commonly used to identify intra-abdominal injuries in adults, is rarely if ever useful in children. The indication for laparotomy in children with trauma is haemodynamic instability despite appropriate volume resuscitation and not the mere presence or absence of intra-abdominal bleeding.

Once the life threatening injuries have been identified, resuscitation and stabilisation commenced, and the lesser injuries identified, then consideration needs to be given as to where definitive care should be given. This may well require the child to be transferred to another facility. Preparation for transfer should include ensuring cardiorespiratory stability, adequate vascular access, gastric decompression and full documentation of both the injuries and therapy.

One of the most underutilised piece of equipment in the management of severe injury is the telephone. It should be used to obtain advice when needed from experts and to ensure good communication between referring and receiving clinicians.

53 Vaginal Discharge and Vulval Irritation

In the newborn infant, the vagina has white mucoid secretions which may last a week or more. The secretions may become tinged with blood a few days after birth. The secretions are due to stimulation of the foetus *in utero* by maternal and placental hormones. The blood staining is due to withdrawal of these hormones after birth. These require no treatment other than reassurance and explanation to the parents.

HISTORY

The presenting symptoms include vulvar itch, soreness, bleeding, urinary symptoms, vaginal discharge, perianal skin soiling or a specific skin lesion. In order to make an aetiological diagnosis, it is important to ask about history of recent respiratory infections, urinary symptoms (including enuresis), medications (especially antibiotics), skin ailments (such as allergy, eczema, psoriasis, seborrhoea), diabetes mellitus, nocturnal perianal itchiness, type of clothing, perfume, deodorants, soap, baths (for example bubble baths) used, diarrhoea and pain on defaecation. Information should also be sought about perineal hygiene and general health of the child.

EXAMINATION

A knowledge of normal anatomy and good examination technique, bright light and a reassuring manner are essential in making the correct diagnosis.

The child is examined in the supine position or in the knee-chest position. The knee-chest position allows a good view of the vagina without resorting to instrumentation.

The structures of importance are the labia majora, labia minora, clitoris, the vaginal vestibule, the hymen, the fossa navicularis and the posterior fouchette (Fig. 4.1). Traction is applied to the labia majora. This allows the hymen to be seen and allows a limited view of the posterior vagina. Simple inspection is all that is require in most cases. A rectal examination is performed to look for a hard foreign body, a normal cervix and pelvic tumours. Vaginoscopy should be reserved for persistent or recurrent vulvovaginitis, bleeding or suspicion of foreign body, neoplasm or congenital anomaly.

Inspect underclothes for evidence of discharge. A general physical examination is also carried out with particular attention to the skin, ears, nose and throat and sexual development.

A sterile medicine dropper filled with saline inserted into the vagina can be used to flush the area and will help with obtaining specimens for bacteriology.

DIAGNOSIS

Important investigations include vaginal swabs, urinalysis, cellotape slide test for worms and pelvic ultrasound or X-ray in exceptional cases.

The causes of vulval irritation and vaginal discharge can be divided into local irritation and infection (local or systemic).

Local Irritation

This may be due to faeces (poor hygiene), tight underwear, especially nylon or lycra, perfumed soaps, bubble bath, and toilet tissue.

Poor hygiene: Children are not by nature hygienic and faecal contamination of the vulvar region occurs easily due to the short perineum, wiping back to front, scratching, and inadequate cleaning after defaecation.

Clothing: Tight, non-absorbable clothing leads to friction and increased heat and sweating which increases the likelihood of inflammation, itching and erythema.

Soaps, bubble baths, tissues (perfumed): These may give rise to local dermatitis because of chemical irritants.

Sandbox play: Children may sit in sandboxes which may be contaminated with animal excreta. Entrapment of sand particles in clothing will cause irritation.

Nappy rash: This has to be distinguished from the systemic skin diseases, such as atopic and seborrheic dermatitis, psoriosis and lichen sclerosis et atrophicus.

Sexual abuse: Non-specific genital complaints including redness, itch or vaginal discharge may be the presenting complaint in sexual abuse. Sensitive questioning of the parent and child may allow this to be recognised and a more formal evaluation to take place.

Infections

Non specific vulvovaginitis: Poor local hygiene leads to a primary vulvitis and a secondary vaginitis. Culture may show a mixture of diphtheroids, staphylococci, streptococci and coliforms.

Candida albicans (thrush): Is often associated with administration of antibiotics, diabetes mellitus, immunodeficiency or oestrogen therapy. The newborn may get oral thrush or vaginitis from the birth canal. Children with atopic or seborrheic dermatitis and napkin rash may have sporadic candida infection.

Threadworms: Are present in 20–30% of cases with vulvar symptoms. The history may reveal nocturnal perianal puritus. Cellotape test will confirm the diagnosis. These patients develop non-specific bacterial vulvovaginitis secondary to scratching.

Specific organisms: These may be associated with infection elsewhere and include Group A Beta haemolytic streptococcus, Streptococcus pneumonia, Haemophilus influenza B and Neiseria meningitidis. Isolation of gonococcus, chlamydia, trichomonas and/or the presence of condylomata suggests the likelihood of sexual abuse if the child is above the age of 2 years as vertical transmission is unlikely after this age.

TREATMENT

1. Tepid baths for 15–30 minutes.
2. Do not use soap.
3. 1% hydrocortisone cream.
4. Wash vulval area bd and pat dry.
5. Hair dryer can be used to dry area.
6. Ideally wash after each bowel movement.
7. Wipe vulva front to back.
8. Cotton underwear.
9. Avoid tight clothes and swimsuits.
10. Administer appropriate antibiotics if necessary.
11. If symptoms are persistent or recurrent and vaginoscopy shows no abnormality, then use topical oestrogen.

54 Persistent Vomiting

Vomiting without diarrhoea is a common symptom. The cause may be trivial or indicate a serious illness.

HISTORY

Age and associated symptoms must be taken into account for arriving at a diagnosis. Other factors that need to be considered are the frequency, forcefulness and the nature of the vomitus, e.g. blood, bile.

In the newborn infant the most common cause is gastric irritation due to swallowed amniotic fluid which may contain vaginal secretions and meconium. Infants with tracheo-oesophageal fistula are mucusy and "spit". Infants with upper gastrointestinal tract obstruction will present with persistent vomiting within the first 48 hours of life with little or no abdominal distension. The vomitus will contain bile if obstruction is below the ampulla of Vater. In lower gastrointestinal obstruction, abdominal distension is the prominent symptom and vomiting occurs later. Systemic infections and raised intracranial pressure may also present with vomiting in the newborn but it is usually not the presenting symptom. Metabolic disorders and adrenogenital disorders may also present with severe vomiting — the diagnosis may be obvious (e.g. ambiguous genitalia) or can be made only after investigations (e.g. serum electrolytes, endocrine investigations).

In the infant, gastro-oesophageal reflux is a frequent cause and may be a nuisance rather than a problem. However, it may be accompanied with severe irritability, failure to thrive, aspiration pneumonia and haematemesis as well as anaemia. In the alert hungry infant below the age of 3 months, projectile vomiting with infrequent stools suggests a diagnosis of pyloric stenosis. In the infant who has been weaned and has severe intermittent colic, intussusception is a likely diagnosis.

Enteric and systemic infections (including urinary tract infection) can present with vomiting at any age and may be accompanied with diarrhoea. Poisoning (lead, toxins, fungi) and inappropriate foods can also cause vomiting at any age. Vomiting due to raised intracranial pressure is often worse in the morning and is frequently accompanied by irritability in infants and headache in older children. Rarer causes in older children include psychological (e.g. birthday party, excitement), diabetes mellitus, migraine and "abdominal epilepsy" — the history may be the clue to the diagnosis in such cases.

EXAMINATION

In acute vomiting, signs of dehydration (depressed fontanelle, loss of skin turgor, dry mouth, sunken eyes, decreased urine output, hypotension), may be present. In chronic vomiting, there is evidence of malnutrition (failure to thrive, anaemia, specific vitamin deficiencies). Other physical findings will depend on aetiology, e.g. neurological signs may be present if there is raised intracranial pressure.

MANAGEMENT

In most cases, acute vomiting is a self-limiting problem and other than ensuring adequate fluid intake, no treatment is indicated. Anti-emetics are of limited value and may cause dystonic reactions. In severe cases, dehydration may result. Such infants require admission to hospital for intravenous fluid therapy and monitoring of serum electrolytes.

Investigations may be needed to make an aetiological diagnosis of vomiting. These will depend on the history and physical examination.

55 Wheezing

Wheezing is a frequent and troublesome symptom in infants and children. It is due to airway obstruction and is a result of air travelling at a high speed through a narrowed segment of the airway. Therefore it can only be produced in the central airway (i.e., first of four or five generations of bronchi) as the airflow is too slow in the periphery of the lung to produce the sound.

HISTORY

In making a diagnosis, the age of onset is helpful. Wheezing present from birth suggests structural tracheal abnormalities (tracheobroncho-malacia) or extrinsic tracheal compression (vascular ring, mediastinal tumour, lung cyst). In infants, it may be the result of mucosal oedema following viral infections (particularly respiratory syncytial virus). These patients manifest other signs of infection of the respiratory tract, namely fever, nasal discharge and cough. The recovery is complete and recurrent attacks are unusual. They do not respond to bronchodilator therapy. Often other members of the family will also give a history of respiratory illness. Recurrent wheezing in infants may be due to aspiration which is seen in gastro-oesophageal reflux (frequent vomiting) and infants with neurological problems who have difficulty in swallowing. Hyperreactive airways in infants can also present with recurrent wheezing but these patients will respond to bronchodilator therapy and have a family history of atopy, hay fever, eczema and asthma. They may also give a history of eczema in early infancy. As 20% of infants with cystic fibrosis also have reactive airways disease, they may be misdiagnosed as having asthma. However the history of poor weight gain and signs of parenchymal lung disease should alert the physician. Infants with bronchopulmonary dysplasia also present with recurrent wheezing as they have a hyper-reactive airway. In infants with history of contact with tuberculosis, extrinsic compression with lymph nodes may present with wheezing.

Foreign body aspiration can sometimes present with a wheeze. In these patients, the wheeze is usually localised and it may be possible to obtain a history of choking before the onset of the symptoms (Fig. 55.1).

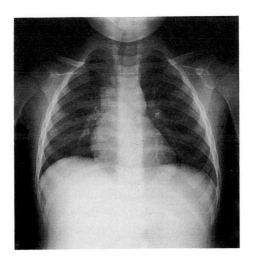

Fig. 55.1 *Foreign Body in bronchus.* Presenting as wheezing and breathlessness. X-ray shows hyperlucent left lung (due to air trapping), flattened diaphragm and shift of mediasternum to right side.

The most common cause of wheezing after infancy is asthma. These patients have a history of recurrent wheezing, cough, which may be particularly worse at night or after exercise. The wheezing may be precipitated by exercise. A family history of atopy or other manifestations of atopy in the patient (eczema, allergic rhinitis) would support the diagnosis. Many children complain of inspiratory difficulty in severe cases. Abdominal pain is common particularly in younger children and presumably is due to the strenuous use of abdominal muscles and the diaphragm.

Respiratory tract infections (particularly mycoplasma) may also present with a wheeze. The diagnosis in these patients is often made after investigations.

Infants with wheezing are sometimes irritable because of hypoxia and have feeding difficulties as the rapid respiratory rate may not permit time for sucking and swallowing.

EXAMINATION

The physical findings will depend upon the severity of the wheezing and the underlying disease process. Most patients have increased respiratory rate (in bronchiolitis it may be as high as 100–120 per minute). In severe cases, there is air hunger and cyanosis may be present. There is flaring of the alae nasi, intercostal and subcostal retractions and evidence of hyperinflation (loss of liver and cardiac dullness, palpable liver). The expiratory phase of breathing is prolonged and wheezes are usually audible. In the most severe cases, breath sounds may be absent as air does not enter the alveoli. Tachycardia and pulsus paradoxus may be present depending upon the severity of the wheezing attack.

MANAGEMENT

All patients with wheezing should have at least one X-ray of the chest as it may help in diagnosing and institution of specific treatment. Other investigations (e.g. airway screening, barium swallow) may be necessary to confirm the diagnosis.

Full blood count will often show eosinophilia in asthma, tropical eosinophilia and other parasitic diseases which may present with wheezing. Allergy skin testing is of limited value in children with wheezing. Tuberculin testing is indicated in patients suspected of having primary tuberculosis.

Pulmonary function testing is valuable in the evaluation of children in whom asthma is suspected. Such tests are useful in assessing the degree of airway obstruction and measuring the response of the airways to inhaled allergens and in assessing the response to bronchodilator therapy. The response to bronchodilator therapy (an increase of 15% in FEV_1) can be used as a diagnostic tool in asthma.

Most children with recurrent wheezing will have asthma. The rest of this chapter describes the management of such patients.

Avoidance of allergens: It is difficult or impractical to avoid exposure to allergens that are difficult to identify. However, it is possible to avoid exposure to certain recognised indoor allergens such as house dust, danders and moulds. Control of house dust in the child's bedroom may ameliorate symptoms in the dust allergic child. Avoidance of damp basements and the application of measures designed to discourage mould growth in the house are useful for the child sensitive to moulds. Other measures include dehumidifiers, air conditioners and air cleaning devices. However the physician should keep in sight that these measures may fail and cause financial hardship to the parents. The patients should avoid tobacco smoke, strong odours such as wet paint and disinfectants, ice cold drinks and rapid changes in temperature and humidity. Maintenance of humidified air is important in dry cold climates in the winter.

The mainstay of treatment of acute asthma is bronchodilator therapy and oxygen. Prophylactic therapy for chronic asthma includes sodium chromoglycate and inhaled corticosteroids.

Every child with asthma should have education in the role of medications and understand the principles of treatment. Children having recurrent attacks should have an asthma action plan in the event of an acute attack.

Index